SCHIZOPHRENIA TREATMENT - THE NEW FACETS

Edited by **Yu-Chih Shen**

Schizophrenia Treatment - The New Facets
http://dx.doi.org/10.5772/62958
Edited by Yu-Chih Shen

Contributors

Sheng-An Lee, Kuo-Chuan Huang, Tse-Yi Wang, Theresa Tsun-Hui Tsao, Anton Loonen, Svetlana A. Ivanova, MariaCristina Turola, Davide Barbieri, Angelo Palazzi, Veronica Pallotta, Luciana Simani, Chiara Tosi, Ombretta Zanardi, Libor Ustohal, Tomas Sverak, Lenka Albrechtova, Marie Hojgrova, Veronika Hublova, Tomas Kasparek, Verónica Juárez Ramos, Wen-Jun Gao, Sarah Monaco, Shiva Singh, Melkaye Melka, Christina Castellani, José Gutiérrez-Fernández, Antonio Sorlozano

Published by InTech

Janeza Trdine 9, 51000 Rijeka, Croatia

Publishing Process Manager Iva Lipovic

Technical Editor SPi Global

Cover InTech Design team

First published December, 2016

Printed in Croatia

Additional hard copies can be obtained from orders@intechopen.com

Schizophrenia Treatment - The New Facets, Edited by Yu-Chih Shen

p. cm.

Print ISBN 978-953-51-2825-0
Online ISBN 978-953-51-2826-7

For EU product safety concerns:
IN TECH d.o.o., Prolaz Marije Krucifikse Kozulić 3, 51000 Rijeka, Croatia,
info@intechopen.com or visit our website at intechopen.com.

Meet the editor

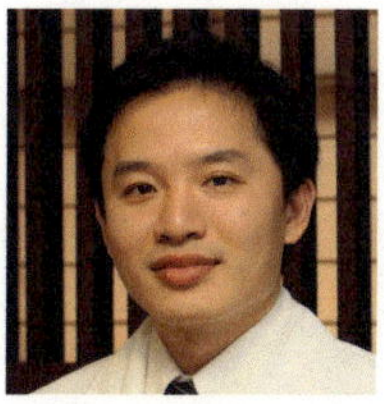

Dr. Yu-Chih Shen is the director of the Department of Psychiatry at Tzu Chi General Hospital, Hualien, Taiwan. He is also an associate professor of Psychiatry and Clinical Psychology at Tzu Chi University, Hualien, Taiwan. Dr. Shen was born in Taiwan in 1976. He graduated from Chung Shan Medical University School of Medicine in 2001. Then he entered the Department of Psychiatry of Tri-Service General Hospital at Taipei, where he completed his 4 years of psychiatric residency training. He moved to Tzu Chi General Hospital in 2005. During the following years, he served as the attending physician (2005–now). He also completed his PhD degree and graduated from Tzu Chi University Institute of Medical Sciences in 2011.

Dr. Shen is actively involved in academic activities. His major research interests are genetic and functional analysis of candidate genes in psychiatric disorder and pharmacogenetic study of psychiatric medication. He has published more than 40 peer-reviewed articles and has worked as a reviewer and an editorial board member for many scientific journals.

Contents

Preface

Schizophrenia treatment has many facets. Among those, other than current available antipsychotic agents and electroconvulsive therapy, this book begins with the glutamatergic and GABAergic hypofunctioning contribute to the schizophrenic symptoms and their current targeted therapeutics. The genetic, epigenetic, and immune etiologies of schizophrenia and their potential targeted therapeutics as approached in this book are interesting because not only the changes in DNA sequence, methylation, and transcriptome contribute to the predisposition of schizophrenia but also the exposure to infectious diseases coupled with a genetic component causes immune system anomaly is presented. Understanding cognitive biases and delusional circuits in schizophrenia is important; several behavioral cognitive therapies working on the reduction and avoidance of these cognitive biases are demonstrating their effectiveness. Advances in schizophrenia treatment followed, including transcranial magnetic stimulation and special sport program, are presented at the book's end. Clearly, schizophrenia treatment will even become a greater topic in the generations to come as new pathophysiologic view and therapy evolve. This book collects some important facets for future comprehensive coverage, as developments abound.

Yu-Chih Shen, MD, PhD
Department of Psychiatry, Tzu Chi General Hospital, Hualien, Taiwan
Department of Psychiatry, School of Medicine, Tzu Chi University, Hualien, Taiwan

Chapter 1

The Convergence of Glutamate and GABA Dysregulation in Schizophrenia

Sarah A. Monaco, Austin A. Coley and Wen-Jun Gao

Additional information is available at the end of the chapter

http://dx.doi.org/10.5772/65870

Abstract

Schizophrenia (SCZ) is a heterogeneous neurodevelopmental disorder that afflicts about 1% of the world population, imposing a huge financial and social burden on the community. Schizophrenia is characterized by three core features, positive (e.g., hallucinations, delusions) and negative symptoms (e.g., emotional blunting, reduced motivation), as well as cognitive impairments (i.e., working memory and attention deficits). Current antipsychotic treatments, which primarily target dopamine receptors, are effective at alleviating positive symptoms. However, dopamine-specific therapies are insufficient to relieve negative symptoms and cognitive impairments, indicating other neuronal systems are involved in SCZ. Evidence for hypofunctioning glutamate and gamma-aminobutyric acid (GABA) transmission in forebrain tissue has continued to culminate as major contributors to the onset of SCZ. Furthermore, recent genetic studies reveal disrupted mutations in neurodevelopmental proteins at glutamatergic and GABAergic synapses that are potentially responsible for the synaptic abnormalities seen in the disorder. Therefore, schizophrenia symptomatology is influenced by interactions of several neurotransmitter systems. In this chapter, we focus on how glutamatergic and GABAergic hypofunctioning contribute to the variety of symptoms presented in SCZ and its etiology. We also review the current treatment options with respect to their mechanism of action, side effects, and limitations and provide perspective of where research should be directed to move forward with treating this debilitating disease.

Keywords: neurodevelopment, glutamate, GABA, negative symptoms, cognitive deficits, treatment, schizophrenia

1. Introduction

Schizophrenia is a chronic mental disorder that afflicts approximately 1.1% of the population worldwide. Patients not only experience physical and mental disabilities, but also impose a large financial burden that consumes an estimated over $60 billion in costs per year, including more than $20 billion in treatment in the United States of America alone.

Schizophrenic patients exhibit an array of clinical symptoms that consist of positive symptoms, negative symptoms, and cognitive impairments. Due to the heterogeneity in symptomatology, this disorder is difficult to diagnose and treat. Typically, the onset of symptoms occurs between adolescence and early adulthood, mostly within the age range of 16–30 years old, occurring in men (average 18) earlier than women (average 25). Cognitive and social deficits are the first symptoms to appear and exacerbate over time. Individuals display a lack of attention, short-term and long-term memory loss, as well as lack of executive functions that include disorganized thoughts and planning. In addition, patients have difficulties communicating ideas and notions, consequently leading to social withdrawal. As the individual gets older, negative symptoms appear, including a blunted affect of normal behavior and feelings. For instance, patients will express a lack in motivation and/or pleasure that often leads to depression and mood swings. Positive symptoms develop later and signify an escalated state of mind and altered reality, such as hallucinations, delusions, and false ideas. The amalgamation of these symptoms persist into adulthood and may perhaps lead to other comorbidities such as attention deficit hyperactive disorder (ADHD), depression, anxiety, aggression, and substance abuse [1].

Unfortunately, schizophrenia is challenging to diagnose due to the various signs and symptoms; however, neuroanatomical evidence displays structural aberrations in specific tissues that assist in characterizing the disorder. For instance, postmortem patients show an overall decrease in brain volume and more specifically reduced cortical gray matter in forebrain tissue, such as the dorsolateral prefrontal cortex (dlPFC), superior temporal gyrus, and limbic areas (i.e., hippocampal formation, anterior cingulate cortex). Other anatomical anomalies include enlarged cerebral ventricles, such as the lateral and third ventricles. Lastly, at the cellular level, there are reports of reduced neuronal number and dendritic spine densities in the hippocampus and dorsolateral prefrontal cortex [2, 3], although this observation appears to be controversial. Nevertheless, numerous studies have confirmed a significant decrease in pyramidal dendritic spines within superficial layers of the prefrontal cortex [2, 4].

The neurophysiological changes are equally as detrimental as the structural changes observed in schizophrenic patients. For example, the most prevailing theories describing the etiology of schizophrenia is the "Dopamine hypothesis," which predicts dopamine imbalances within the mesocortical and mesolimbic pathways underlie schizophrenia pathology. Specifically, dopamine deficiency from mesocortical projecting neurons to the prefrontal cortex results in "hypostimulation" of D1-receptor neurons that contribute to the negative symptoms and cognitive impairments. In contrast, an excess of dopamine to the prefrontal cortex and striatum from mesolimbic dopamine pathways induces "hyperstimulation" of D2-receptor neurons, responsible for the positive symptoms [5]. Therefore, current treatments target dopamine receptors, but leave other pathophysiological mechanisms untargeted. Typical and atypical antipsychotics, such as haloperidol and clozapine, respectively, block D2-receptors to alleviate psychotic symptoms. However, dopamine-specific targeted therapy is insufficient to relieve other aspects of the disease; therefore, additional neuronal systems are likely involved.

In recent years, evidence has linked glutamatergic and GABAergic systems to the pathology of schizophrenia. An emerging hypothesis of schizophrenia suggests that N-methyl-D-aspartate (NMDA) receptor hypofunction plays a major role in the dysregulation of GABAergic transmission, thereby contributing to the symptoms [6]. In this chapter, we discuss the structure and function of NMDA and gamma-aminobutyric acid (GABA) receptors, including the effects of genetic abnormalities on them and their associated posttranslational modifications and signal transduction pathways. We will also include the reviewed literature describing the multiple neuronal subtypes and circuits involved in schizophrenia and potential therapeutic options.

2. Glutamate hypothesis of schizophrenia

Glutamate is an excitatory neurotransmitter that can act on four major classes of receptors, which are either metabotropic or ionotropic. Metabotropic receptors are G-protein coupled receptors. Metabotropic glutamate receptors are composed of mGluR1-8 subunits and have seven transmembrane segments that are connected to heterotrimeric G proteins. The remaining three classes are ionotropic receptors, or ion-gated channels, that consist of NMDA, AMPA, and kainite receptors, which are readily distinguished by agonists, antagonists, kinetics, and permeability. Ionotropic glutamate receptors are composed of a tetramer of four subunits, with each representative monomer consisting of three transmembrane segments, a large extracellular glutamate-binding domain, and a cytosolic loop that lines the channel pore (**Figure 1**).

NMDA receptor hypofunction has long been proposed as one of the major hypothesis for the pathophysiology of schizophrenia [6]. NMDA receptors are highly abundant within the forebrain and are responsible for regulating a variety of neuronal pathways; theoretically, damage to the glutamatergic system could underlie many pathologies of the central nervous system. Accordingly, there is an overwhelming amount of evidence illustrating that NMDA receptor dysfunction contributes to the neurophysiology associated with schizophrenia [6, 7]. For instance, in postmortem subjects with schizophrenia, disruptive mutations of NMDA receptor subunits were revealed in the prefrontal cortex, hippocampus, and thalamus [8, 9]. Furthermore, it is well established that administering noncompetitive NMDA receptor antagonists such as phencyclidine (PCP), MK-801 (also known as Dizocilpine), and ketamine can mimic the pathophysiology and behavioral attributes of schizophrenia [10–12]. Therefore, treatments that target to improve NMDA receptor function demonstrate an alleviation of

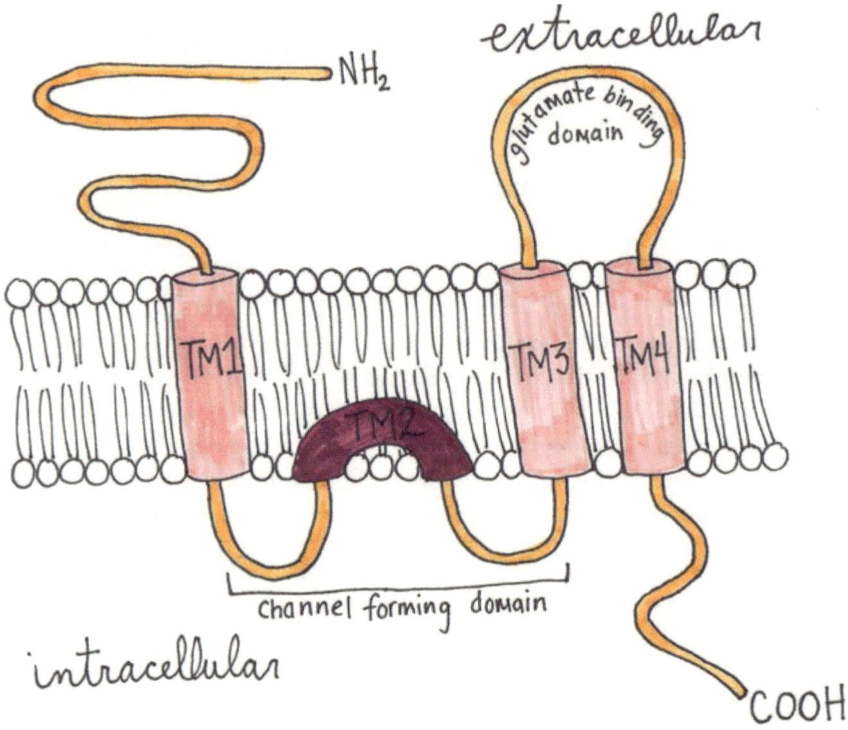

Figure 1. Illustration of prototypic ionotropic receptor subunit. A subunit consists of a large extracellular N-terminus domain, a membrane spanning segment (TM1), a segment that partially enters the membrane (TMII), a glutamate-binding domain, two more membrane spanning segments, and an intracellular c-terminus.

schizophrenic symptoms [13, 14]. Finally, genes implicated in schizophrenia have strong associations with NMDA receptor regulation [15–17].

3. The NMDA receptor structure and function

NMDA receptors are typically located on excitatory glutamatergic synapses, although present in many cell types (i.e., GABAergic neurons, dopaminergic neurons, etc.). NMDA receptors are responsible for synaptic plasticity and cortical development, as well as cognitive processes such as learning and working memory [18]. NMDA receptors are a heterotetrameric complex that consists of an obligatory homodimer of NR1 and homodimers or heterodimers of either combination of NR2A-D or NR3A-D subunits (**Figure 2**). The NMDA channel is voltage-dependent and ligand-gated, and highly permeable to Na^+, K^+, and Ca^{2+}, causing depolarization of a cell and subsequent excitation and activation of intracellular signaling pathways. Although NR1 subunits are required for NMDA receptor function, NR2/NR3 subunits are specialized and critical for functional diversity such as calcium permeability, decay time, open channel time, and pharmacology sensitivity. In addition, NR1 and NR2 subunits

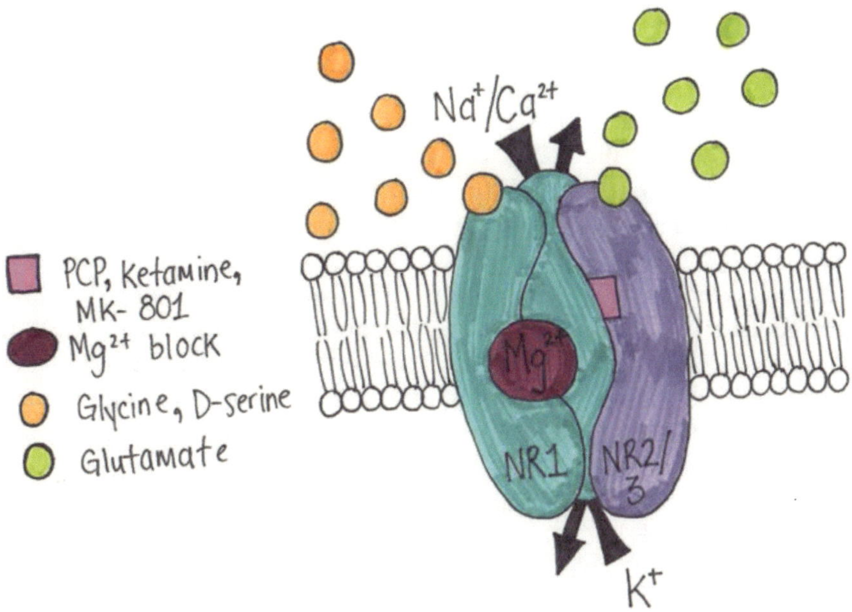

Figure 2. Schematic diagram depicting a NMDA receptor complex. Glutamate binds at NR2/NR3 complex and co-agonist glycine or $_D$-serine binds at NR1 complex. Upon depolarization, Mg^{2+} is removed. NMDA receptor permeates Na^+ and Ca^+ influx and K^+ efflux upon activation. Binding sites for PCP, ketamine, and MK801 are included (Figure was modified from Snyder et al. [6] and Cioffi et al. [14]).

contain distinct sites that bind glycine, PCP, and Mg^{2+} that modulate the activity of NMDA receptors (**Figure 2**).

4. The NMDA receptor development

Developmentally, there is an NR2B- to NR2A-subunit switch that occurs from childhood-to-adulthood in most brain regions that facilitate synaptic maturation [19]. NR2B protein expression levels are highly abundant during early development and decline into adulthood; in contrast, NR2A levels begin low and rise in adult. Both subunits are essential for prefrontal synaptic plasticity and function; however, NR2B plays a more dominant role. For instance, in the prefrontal cortex, NR2B levels remain high into adulthood and are important for working memory function [20, 21]. NR2B-containing NMDA receptors play a major role in calcium (Ca^+) influx at the postsynaptic membrane, as NR2B receptors have slower kinetics, thus a slower decay time compared to NR2A-containing NMDA receptors. This indicates that NR2B receptors conduct a large amount of Ca^+ and Na^+ due to the prolonged open channel state. Although NR2B is essential for cognition processes within the adult, an overabundance may be hazardous due to the significant increase in Ca^+ conductance that could lead to excitotoxicity and neuronal death [21]. Therefore, NR2B/NR2A composition during development is extremely critical for normal synaptic maturation.

5. NMDA receptor dysregulation and hypofunction in schizophrenia

A major finding discovered by functional imaging studies was reduced activity in the dorsolateral prefrontal cortex (dlPFC) in patients with schizophrenia. The overall reduction in neuronal activity in the dlPFC could explain the cognitive deficits and negative symptoms. There is consensus that NMDA receptor hypofunction is strongly associated with the pathophysiology of schizophrenia. In human studies, single-photon emission computed tomography (SPECT) shows "hypofrontality" patients suffering from schizophrenia [22]. Furthermore, there are genetic implications that show single-nucleotide polymorphisms (SNPs) and a reduction in NR1 protein and mRNA in the dorsolateral prefrontal cortex in postmortem subjects of schizophrenia [9, 23]. Additionally, exome sequencing of patients with schizophrenia also displays disruptive mutations in genes that encode NMDAR subunits and NMDA receptor-associate scaffolding proteins, such as PSD-95 and SAP102 [24, 25]. These findings would suggest a lack of and/or function at the postsynaptic membrane of excitatory synapses that could be responsible for the cellular phenotypes of the disorder.

Noncompetitive NMDA receptor antagonists such as PCP, MK-801, and ketamine have been extensively used to study the symptoms associated with schizophrenia in both human subjects and animal models [26]. Indeed, these studies have shown to mimic the effects of schizophrenia, corroborating the glutamatergic hypofunction hypothesis. Individually, PCP induces psychotic symptoms in healthy humans that resemble schizophrenic-like behavior; MK-801 elicits positive and negative symptoms; and lastly ketamine administration was shown to imitate the positive, negative, and cognitive deficits seen in schizophrenia [11]. In rats, NMDA receptor antagonists cause deficits in working memory, executive functions, and enhanced locomotor activity [27].

6. High-risk genes implicated in schizophrenia

High-risk genes associated with schizophrenia such as DISC1, dysbindin, neuregulin, COMT, and G72/G30 genes, responsible for neurodevelopment, neuronal growth, and migration, have all shown to be involved in NMDA dysfunction leading to schizophrenia [15]. The most prominent of the genes is Disrupted in *schizophrenia* 1 (DISC1), which acts as a scaffolding protein involved in the formation of protein complexes important in neurodevelopment, microtubule network dynamics and axonal elongation [28, 29]. Despite the controversy and debate [16, 30], evidence shows that schizophrenic patients contain DISC1-SNPs that cause a decrease in DISC1-interacting protein expression levels, such as NMDA receptors. In DISC1 animal models, mice with point mutations in the gene or truncated forms of DISC1 display molecular, cellular, and behavioral phenotypes that are analogous to schizophrenia. DISC1 is especially susceptible to mutations due to environmental stressors during neurodevelopment that may lead to the pathogenesis of the disorder [31, 32].

7. Other factors affecting NMDA receptor function

Environmental factors during development, such as infection, drug use, parental age, prenatal and early postnatal or childhood stress, have all been linked to the emergence of schizophrenia [33]. In addition, NMDA receptor function is susceptible to the latter environmental risk factors during adolescence, potentially contributing to the onset of the disorder [6, 33, 34]. This could be due to an alteration in NMDA receptor gene expression, as major transcriptional factors such as the cAMP response element binding protein (CREB) are extremely sensitive to environmental stimuli [35]. Previous studies describe that neurodevelopment in the prefrontal cortex is altered in patients with schizophrenia due to a substantial increase in synaptic elimination of glutamatergic excitatory synapses [36].

NMDA receptors are also influenced by posttranslational modifications such as ubiquitination, palmitoylation, and phosphorylation [34]. NMDA receptor phosphorylation is responsible for regulating receptor trafficking, stabilization, kinetics of the channel, and kinase activation. These processes are important for synaptic plasticity during neurodevelopment and if dysregulated could be highly responsible for the pathologies of schizophrenia [7]. NMDA receptor subunits are phosphorylated at serine/threonine and tyrosine residues, providing substrate sites for kinases such as Src family of kinases (SFK), casein kinase 2 (CK2), cAMP-dependent protein kinase A (PKA), cyclin-dependent kinase 5 (Cdk5), protein kinase C (PKC), and Ca^{2+}/calmodulin-dependent protein kinase II (CaMKII) [37–40].

Other modification processes such as palmitoylation and ubiquitination have also been directly linked to schizophrenia [41]. There is evidence of NMDA receptor dysregulation due to anomalous modifications that could potentially lead to neuropsychiatric disorders. Palmitoylation is a process that allows the covalent attachment of palmitate group to the cysteine residues of proteins that are facilitated via thioester bonds. Recently, it has shown to be involved in regulating NR2 subunit trafficking during neurodevelopment and synaptic plasticity [42] and is altered in a mouse model of 22q11.2 deletion syndrome. Ubiquitination is a process involved in the targeting and removal of proteins and is responsible for regulating NMDA receptors degradation during development. Specifically, subunits such as NR1 and NR2B undergo polyubiquitination at the synapse [41]. Nonetheless, palmitoylation and ubiquitination require further investigation in its role in NMDA receptor regulation and potential implication in schizophrenia.

8. Intracellular mechanisms affecting NMDA receptor function

Selective intracellular signal transduction pathways, such as the AKT-GSK3β pathway, at excitatory glutamatergic synapses regulate NMDA receptor functions, and are associated with high-risk genes involved in schizophrenia. AKT, also known as protein kinase B, is a serine/threonine kinase involved in neuronal plasticity, migration, protein synthesis, and cell death [43, 44]. Glycogen synthase kinase 3β (GSK3β) is also a serine/threonine kinase that is downstream of AKT and upstream of beta-catenin [45]. Moreover, GSK3β knockdown leads to a reduction in NMDA receptor current [46]. AKT phosphorylation is a negative regulator of GSK3β activity; similarly, GSK3β phosphorylation induces beta-catenin degradation. High-risk genes such as DISC1, dysbindin and NRG1 are all modulators of the AKT-GSK3β signaling pathway [34]. For instance, reduced DISC1 protein expression causes a decrease in AKT phosphorylation, and thus an increase in GSK3β activity [47]. In addition, reducing GSK3β activity can alleviate the behavioral impairments observed in DISC1 mouse models [48, 49]. These data suggest a link between high-risk schizophrenia genes and intracellular pathways, such as the AKT-GSK3B signaling pathway, that regulate neuronal plasticity. Theoretically, it can be assumed that the high-risk schizophrenia genes would affect the AKT-GSK3β signaling pathway, and thus cause NMDA receptor dysfunction, leading to aberrant neuronal systems that are responsible for the positive, negative, and cognitive symptoms observed in schizophrenia.

9. Drug treatment that targets NMDA receptors

Typically, drug treatment for schizophrenia patients consists of antipsychotics, such as clozapine, that target D2 receptors to relieve the positive symptoms. However, a significant portion of schizophrenia subjects do not respond well to D2 antagonists; moreover, the negative and cognitive impairments are barely affected by treatment with antipsychotic drugs. As a result, medical professionals are testing new pharmacological agents that target NMDA receptors as a therapeutic option. Due to the observed glutamate hypofunction impairment in patients, investigative studies have focused on the enhancement of NMDA receptor function. Therefore, high doses of glycine agonists (60 g/day) that act upon the glycine$_B$ modulatory site are used to increase NMDA receptor function [13]. These agonists have been shown to modestly improve the negative and positive symptoms of schizophrenia and are currently being utilized as an adjunctive treatment to primary therapy with D2 antagonists. An alternative option is to target the glycine transporter-1 (GlyT-1) with the selective inhibitor, sarcosine, to increase glycine availability for NMDA receptor binding [14]. Sarcosine administered at 2 g/day have shown to improve negative and cognitive symptoms of schizophrenia. Other drugs include *d*-Serine and *d*-amino acid oxidase (DAAO) inhibitors to increase *d*-Serine availability, as it is considered a co-agonist to NR1. The effects of the inhibitor were shown to alleviate negative and cognitive impairments in patients when administered at high doses (>2 g/day) and as a supplement to antipsychotic treatments [14]. Kynurenine aminotransferase II (KATII) inhibitors are used to block kynurenic acid (an endogenous antagonist at the NR1 glycine$_B$ site) used to improve negative symptoms. NR2 subtype selective modulators are still under drug development and could prove beneficial to a neurological disorder, such as schizophrenia. Other pharmacological drugs available that affect glutamate transmission are utilized to target AMPA receptors, mGlu5 receptors, and NMDA receptors on GABAergic interneurons. However, many of these new therapeutic interventions are still in clinical trials, whether they are more effective than the typical and atypical D2-related antipsychotic drugs remains to be determined.

http://dx.doi.org/10.5772/65870

10. Glutamate-GABA association in schizophrenia

It is theorized that NMDA dysfunction in neuronal subtypes of GABAergic and dopaminergic neurons collectively contribute to the neuropathologies of schizophrenia. More specifically, investigators speculate that NMDA receptor hypofunction occurs on GABA interneurons (see **Figure 1** in [6]). Glutamatergic neurons have direct interaction with GABA interneurons, such as basket and chandelier cells, within the cortico-limbic circuitry. These interneurons are responsible for suppressing output from glutamate-releasing pyramidal cells, and due to recurrent collaterals from the two cell types, causes an inhibitory feedback loop. However, if GABAergic activity were suppressed, due to NMDAR dysfunction, it would lead

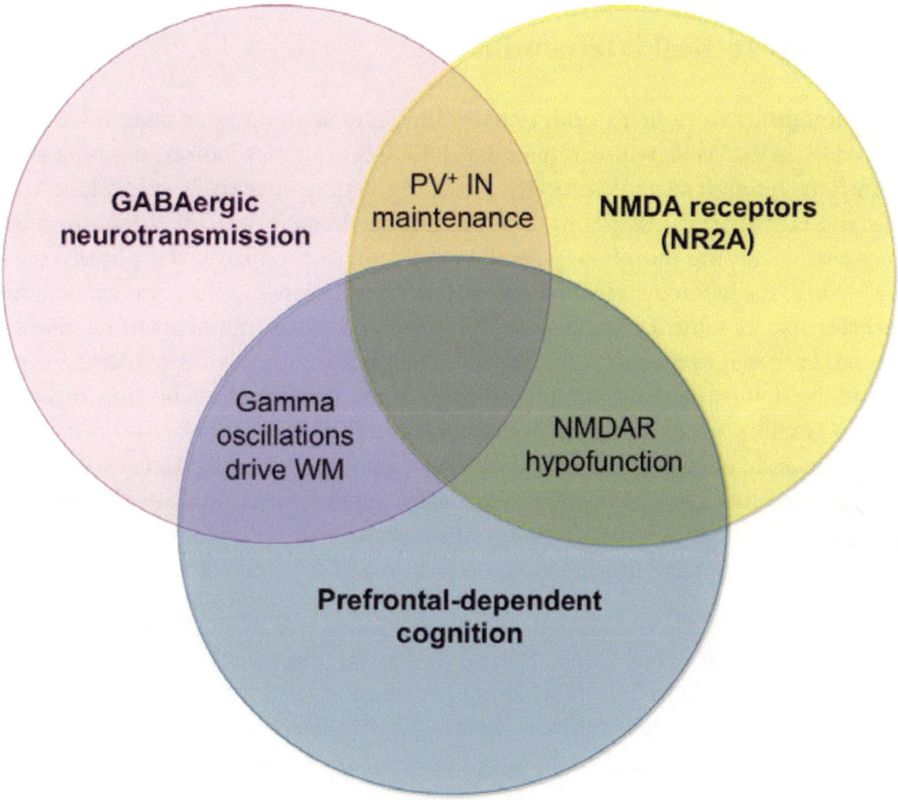

Figure 3. Cross-connections between NMDA receptors, GABAergic neurotransmission, and PFC-dependent cognition. PFC persistent neuronal firing is the foundation of working memory with NMDA receptor activity playing a substantial role in this process [50, 51]. NMDA antagonism in conscious behaving monkeys impairs prefrontal-dependent working memory [52] and induces cognitive impairments in healthy human subjects [11, 53–56], demonstrating a parallel between NMDA hypofunctioning and cognition deficits. This 'online' persistent neural activity is critical for working memory, which is not only NMDAR-dependent, but also requires fast and synchronous inhibition of prefrontal pyramidal neuronal networks by GABAergic interneurons. GABAergic neurotransmission ultimately drives working memory function through the shaping and synchronization of pyramidal cell output. PV cortical interneurons are especially fundamental for generating fast gamma oscillations, which has been demonstrated in humans to be necessary for proper working memory [57]. NMDARs and GABAergic interneurons are interrelated because NMDA receptors play a large role in the maturation [58] and maintenance of interneurons, especially the NR2A subunit [59].

to disinhibition of pyramidal neurons and excessive firing within the cortico-limbic circuit. Physiologically, the excitotoxicity could have multiple effects on circuitry such as changes in membrane potential, receptor desensitization, or cell death. These results would have a twofold effect; first, the GABAergic downregulation would lead to negative symptoms and cognitive deficits. And second, the resulting excess glutamate release of cortico-pyramidal neurons could activate dopaminergic systems that lead to positive symptoms and further cognitive impairments. The glutamate-GABA systems in the forebrain, especially prefrontal cortex, are intertwined to produce prefrontal-dependent cognitive function, as proposed in **Figure 3**. Still, how these two systems interact to induce phenotypes and symptoms in schizophrenia remains to be determined.

11. GABAergic cortical interneurons

Cortical interneurons were first documented with Golgi staining by Santiago Ramón y Cajal and referred to as the "cells with short axons" [60]. Cortical interneurons are typically distinguished by four common attributes: locally projecting, aspiny or sparsely spiny dendrites, small cell soma, and GABAergic. Interneurons exhibit a large diversity and are categorized based on several features including morphology, connectivity, neurochemistry, and physiology [60–62] (**Figure 4**). Due to the heterogeneity of this neuronal population, interneurons can fall into more than one category, showing a great degree of overlap; therefore, interneurons fall more along a spectrum rather than into distinct subgroups. Although this group is very diverse, axonal arborization and the downstream target domain plays a major role in classification and can reveal a lot about a circuitry's function. Essentially, where and how an interneuron synapses onto a target cell ultimately effects neuronal output and therefore function [61], is an essential question for cortical function. Interneurons are crucial for synchronizing and shaping the excitatory activity of pyramidal cells to form a 'task-specific microcircuit' for a particular brain region [61]; the prefrontal cortex contains this microcircuit specialized for working memory [62].

Three common GABAergic neocortical interneurons that will be highlighted and addressed in this chapter are neurochemically defined based on the calcium-binding proteins they express: calbindin (CB), calretinin (CR), and parvalbumin (PV) neurons. Calbindin interneurons (also referred to as somatostatin) makeup ~30% of the cortical interneuronal population and are generally characterized as having either small basket or Martinotti morphology. Commonly, small basket cells target proximal dendrites or the cell soma and electrophysiologically display regular-spiking non-pyramidal (RSNP) activity. Martinotti interneurons exhibit a burst-spiking non-pyramidal (BSNP) firing phenotype and target distal dendrites. Calretinin interneurons are the least prevalent (~15%) and stereotypically have small bipolar morphology. These interneurons target proximal dendrites and also other GABAergic interneurons having either RSNP or BSNP firing. Parvalbumin interneurons are fast-spiking cells and neurochemically the largest group, making up half of the interneuronal population in the cortex. PV interneurons target all along a pyramidal cell, with large basket cells at the proximal dendrites/soma, nest cells at the soma, and chandelier cells targeting the axon initial segment. For the remainder of this section, we will focus on parvalbumin chandelier cells

http://dx.doi.org/10.5772/65870

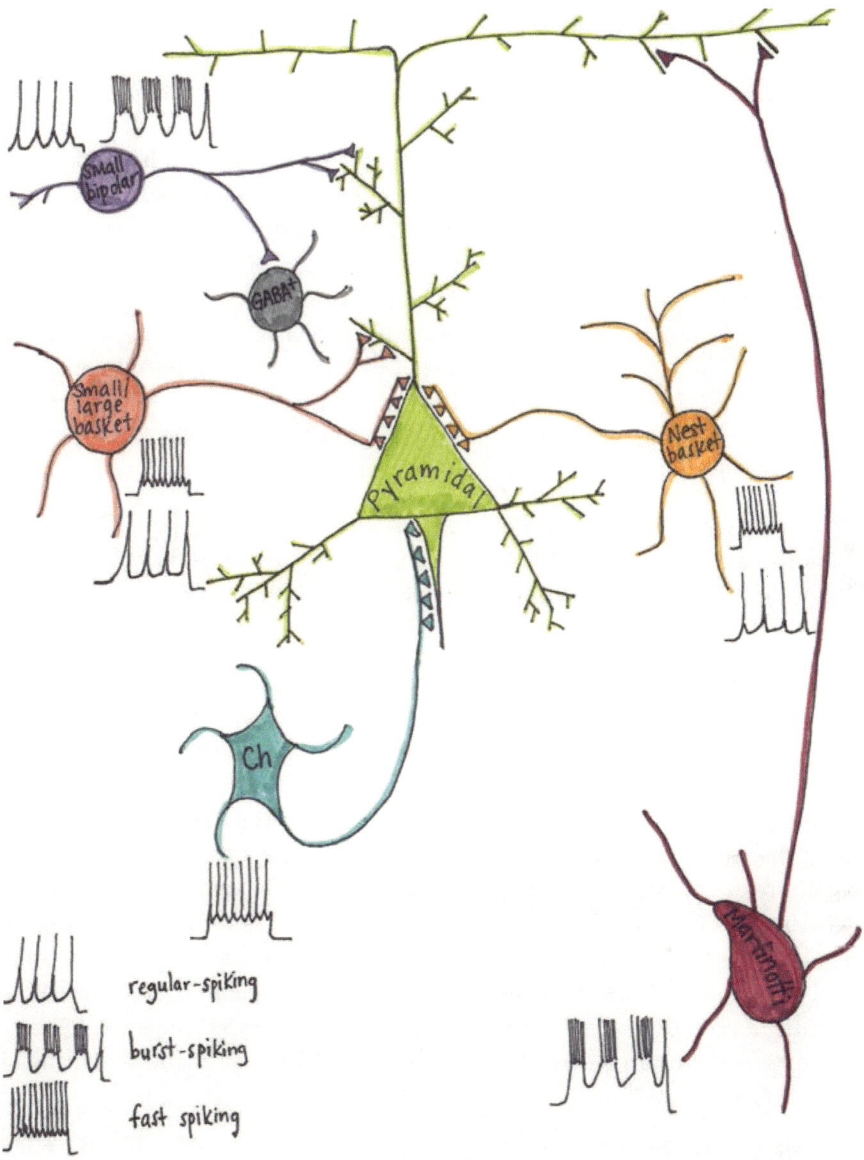

Figure 4. Cortical interneuron connectivity and firing patterns categorized by calcium-binding neurochemical markers. Calretinin small bipolar cells target proximal dendrites and other GABAergic interneurons. Calbindin neurons, small basket cells, and Martinotti cells, target proximal dendrites/soma and distal dendrites. Parvalbumin interneurons are fast-spiking and are further classified into large basket, nest basket, and chandelier (Ch) cells. Large basket cells target proximal dendrites and the soma. Nest basket cells target the cell soma and chandelier cells synapse on the axon initial segment (Modified from Lewis et al. [62]).

since these are the interneurons known to play a major role in prefrontal cortex-dependent working memory and also have been implicated in the pathophysiology of neuropsychiatric disorders such as schizophrenia [60, 62].

12. GABA receptor classification and structure

GABA receptors respond to the ligand GABA, which is the main inhibitory neurotransmitter in the mammalian central nervous system. GABAergic neurons are therefore important for modulating neuronal activity throughout the brain and spinal cord [63–70]. The enzyme L-glutamic acid decarboxylase (GAD) synthesizes GABA in presynaptic terminals through the conversion of glutamate to GABA. GABA is then stored in vesicles waiting for release following neuronal activation [67]. Extracellular GABA can bind to either postsynaptic or extrasynaptic receptors located on presynaptic neurons, leading to hyperpolarization of the target cell [69]. Postsynaptic receptor activation mediates phasic inhibition, whereas extrasynaptic activation mediates a tonic inhibitory state [65, 69]. To remove extracellular GABA in the synaptic cleft, GABA transporters located on the presynaptic terminal and glial cells regulate neurotransmitter uptake; this process is extremely important to retain a balanced circuitry and prevent over inhibition [67].

GABA receptors are classified into two groups, $GABA_A$ and $GABA_B$, with $GABA_C$ receptors recently categorized as a subtype of $GABA_A$ rather than their own distinct class. Receptor characterization is based on structural, biochemical, modulatory, and physiological differences [67–70].

$GABA_A$ receptors are ionotropic chloride channels, conducting fast inhibitory neurotransmission, in which a ligand (i.e., GABA) binds and directly induces pore opening [67, 69]. $GABA_A$ receptors are members of a much larger group referred to as the Cys-loop ligand-gated ion channel superfamily, which also encompasses nicotinic acetylcholine receptors (nAChRs), glycine receptors, and 5-hydroxytryptamine type-3 (5-HT_3) receptors [65, 68–70]. The diverse pharmacology displayed by $GABA_A$ receptors sets them apart from the rest of the family and is clinically relevant targets for anticonvulsant, anxiolytic, and sedative drugs [65, 69]. Typically, $GABA_A$ receptors are heteropentameric structures composed of five different subunits (α1-6, β1-3, ϒ1-3 (ϒ2S, ϒ2L), ϱ1-3, δ, ε, θ, and π), each containing four transmembrane domains (TM1-4) (**Figures 5** and **6**). Five out of twenty-one available subunits comprise the complex, forming a pore from the TM2 segments [67–70]. The top three most common structural compositions in the brain are α1β2γ2, α2β3γ2, and α3β3γ2, with the likely stoichiometry of 2α:2β:1γ [65, 67, 69].

Benzodiazepines potentiate the inhibitory effects of GABA by allosterically altering the receptor and increasing its affinity for GABA [67]. Benzodiazepine-insensitive receptors are formed when the γ subunit is replaced by δ, ε, or π [69]. Rho (ϱ) subunits are unique because these subunits predominately co-assemble together to form homo- and hetero-oligomers. Previously, ϱ oligomers were classified as $GABA_C$ receptors, but more recently are considered a subclass of $GABA_A$ receptors. Even though $GABA_A$ and $GABA_C$ receptors are structurally very similar to one another, these receptors formally fell into two different groups based on their differential pharmacology and physiology [69, 70]. A major difference between the A and C subtypes are that $GABA_A$ receptors are selectively blocked by bicuculline and modulated by benzodiazepines, steroids, and barbiturates. $GABA_C$ receptors are not sensitive to the same drugs, but rather are blocked by 1,2,5,6-tetrahydropyridin-4-yl) methylphosphinic

http://dx.doi.org/10.5772/65870

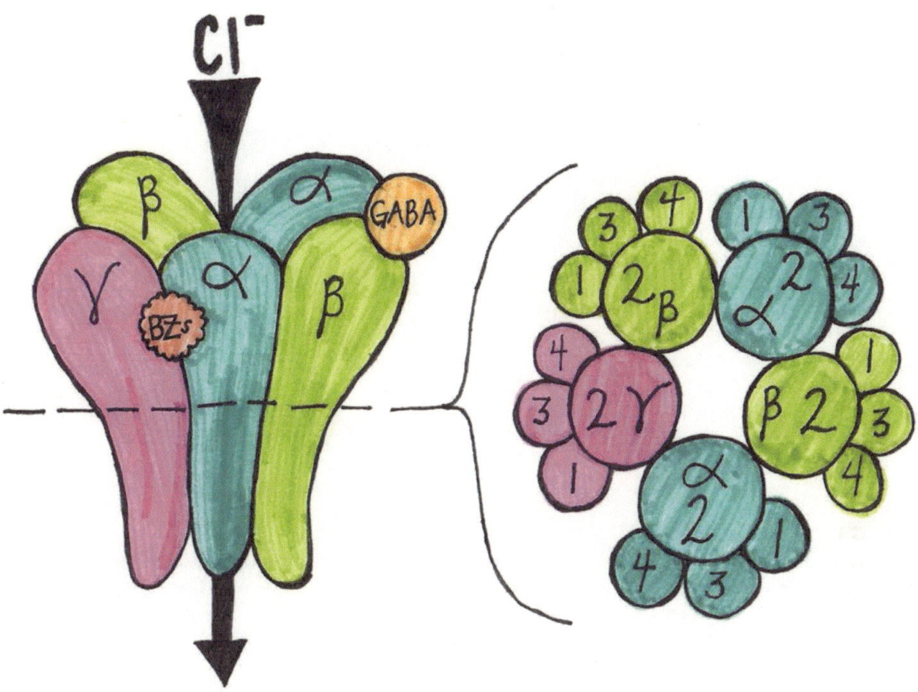

Figure 5. $GABA_A$ receptor structure and cross-section. $GABA_A$ receptors contain five subunits, typically in the ratio of 2α:2β:1γ, with the transmembrane domain 2 (TM2) forming the chloride-permeable pore. Each subunit consists of four hydrophobic transmembrane domains with the N- and C- terminus facing the extracellular side. The GABA binding site is located at the interface between α and β subunit, while the benzodiazepine (BZs) binding site sits at the junction between α and γ. GABA binding triggers channel opening, allowing inward chloride ion flux, whereas benzodiazepine binding potentiates the GABA-induced chloride influx [65, 69] (Modified from Jacob et al. [65] and Vithlani et al. [69]).

acid (TPMPA) and activated by Z-4-amniobut-2-enoic acid [cis-aminocrotonic acid (CACA)]. Additionally, $GABA_C$ receptors exhibit a higher sensitivity to GABA, conduct less current, have longer channel opening times, and desensitize slower in the presence of an agonist. $GABA_C$ receptors, however, are no longer classified as a separate division, but are now considered a $GABA_A$-ϱ subclass because they are exclusively constructed of ϱ subunits [70].

$GABA_B$ receptors are metabotropic Ca^{2+} or K^+ channels, conducting slow inhibitory neurotransmission, in which a ligand (i.e., GABA) binds and indirectly induces pore opening through G-protein coupling activation and second messenger signaling [64, 67, 68] (**Figure 7**). Functional $GABA_B$ receptors exist as heterodimers composed of one $GABA_{B(1)}$ (1a-g) and one $GABA_B$ subunit [70]. The $GABA_{B(1)}$ subunit binds to GABA and is mandatory for functional receptors, whereas the $GABA_{B2}$ subunit is responsible for G-protein coupling and signaling. The most prevalent $GABA_B$ isoforms are $GABA_{B(1a)}$ and $GABA_{B(1b)}$, which are highly conserved across species. Other isoforms, 1c-g, have also been identified, but are either species-specific or do not exist naturally [64]. Baclofen, clinically used as a muscle relaxant, stimulates $GABA_B$ receptors, which are otherwise insensitive to drugs that modulate the $GABA_A$ receptors [67].

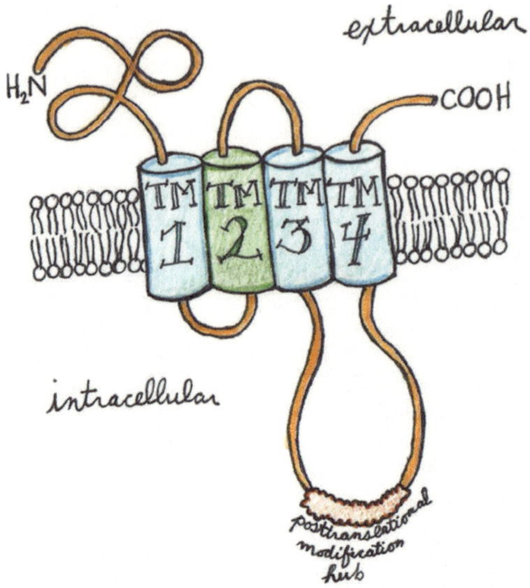

Figure 6. $GABA_A$ receptor transmembrane topology. Each subunit consists of four transmembrane domains. The N- and C-terminus lie on the extracellular side, with the N-terminus being the site of action for several drugs. A large intracellular domain exists between TM3 and TM4, providing a hub for a majority of the protein-protein interactions as well as posttranslational modifications (palmitoylation, ubiquitination, phosphorylation) [65, 69].

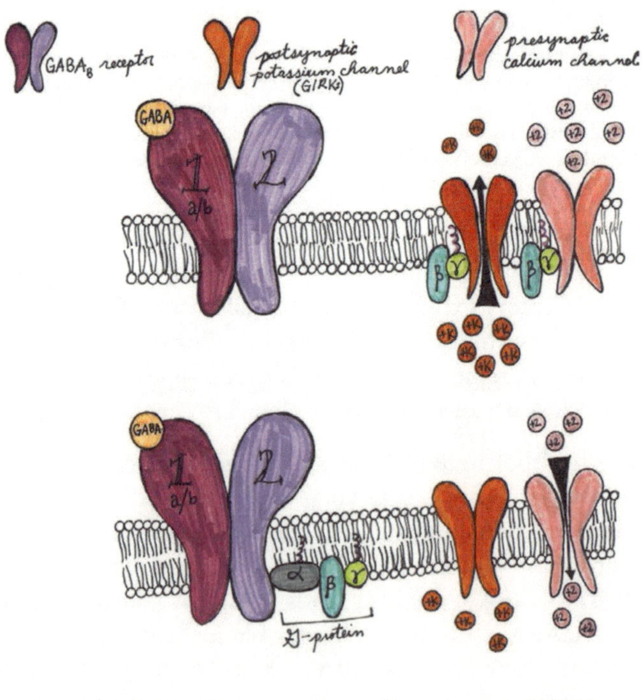

Figure 7. $GABA_B$ receptor structure. $GABA_B$ receptors are heterodimers composed of either a 1a or 1b subunit and a mandatory 2 subunit. $GABA_B$ receptors are G-protein coupled and are activated by the ligand GABA, which binds to the 1 subunit. Following GABA ligand binding, G-protein activation induces opening of postsynaptic potassium channels and closing of presynaptic calcium channels, hyperpolarizing the target cell (Modified from Emson [64]).

13. Distribution

$GABA_A$ subunit expression has been well characterized in the rat brain [66]. Several subunits exhibit broad expression throughout the nervous system, fluctuating across development and regions. However, a few subunits demonstrate regional or cell-type specificity. For example, $\alpha 6$ subunit is exclusively expressed in cerebellar granule cells and the ϱ subunit is largely restricted to the retina. Peripheral expression of $GABA_A$ receptors has been demonstrated in the liver, smooth airway muscles, the lung, immune cells, and the intestines [68]. $GABA_B$ receptors are localized in the striatum, brainstem, thalamus, hippocampus, cerebellum, and cortex. The 1b subunit is the most prevalently expressed across all brains regions, except for the striatum in which the 1a subunit is the most abundant [64].

14. Parvalbumin interneurons and the prefrontal cortex

The prefrontal cortex (PFC) is the neuroanatomical hub for executive functions such as working memory, which can be metaphorically thought of as the brain's blackboard [21, 71]. Incoming stimuli are transiently stored, manipulated, updated, and guide goal-directed behavior [72]. Working memory is dependent on prefrontal circuitry involving the unique balance between pyramidal Delay excitatory neurotransmission and GABAergic interneuronal inhibition [57, 62, 71]. Excitatory Delay cells become activated upon presentation of a salient cue and sustain neuronal activity throughout a delay period, essentially 'remembering' the cue, and allowing an appropriate response. For instance, **Figure 8** represents an

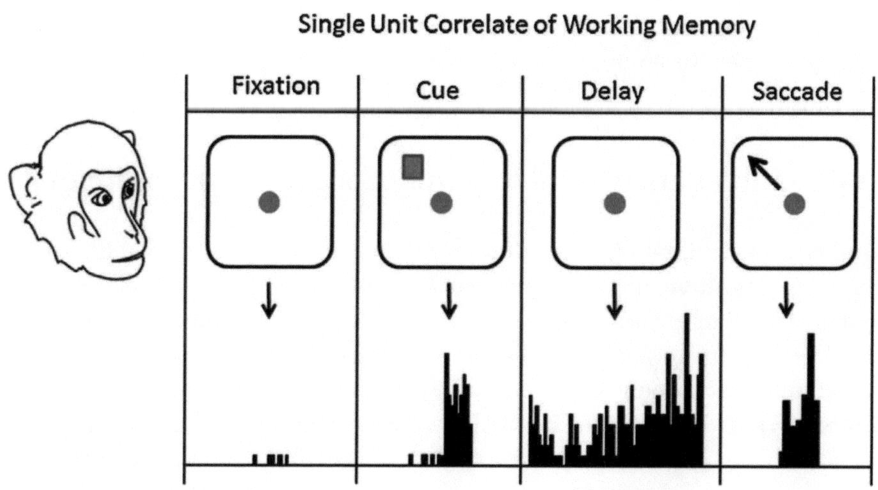

Figure 8. Single unit electrophysiological activity of a Delay cell in the primate DLPFC during a working memory task. The onset of Delay cell activity is triggered by the presence of relevant stimuli, or a cue. In the absence of a visual cue, Delay cells persistently fire during the delay period and allow for the generation of a goal-directed response (e.g., saccade). The sustained neuronal firing during the delay period is hypothesized to be the neural correlate of working memory and depends on both excitatory pyramidal activity as well as fast-spiking GABAergic interneurons in the DLPFC [21, 71, 73, 74] (Modified from Monaco et al. [21]).

example of single unit prefrontal Delay cell activity in the primate dorsolateral prefrontal cortex (DLPFC) during an oculomotor delayed-response task. In this working memory task, subjects are trained to fix their gaze at the center. A single cue is presented somewhere in the 360° perimeter, followed by a brief delay period in which the cue is absent. After the delay period, an appropriate response would be an eye saccade in the direction that the cue was first presented.

Working memory, the sustained neuronal activity that occurs during the delay, is not only dependent on prefrontal pyramidal cells, but also fast-spiking GABAergic interneurons [57, 62, 71]. Pharmacological evidence supports the importance of fast-spiking interneurons in the DLPFC for working memory function. Administration of a $GABA_AR$ antagonist, bicuculline, lead to impaired mnemonic tuning during an oculomotor delayed-response task. Therefore, working memory, particularly sustained neuronal activity during the delay period, depends on $GABA_A$ receptors. Furthermore, GABAergic hypofunctioning in the DLPFC partly contributes to working memory deficits [62, 75]. GABAergic neuronal activity and its role in working memory function are also connected to gamma oscillations. Gamma oscillations, which fall in the band range between 30 and 60 Hz, are required for working memory function. A research study conducted in 2003 reported that gamma band oscillations increased proportionally with working memory load [57, 62, 76]. More specifically, fast-spiking PV interneurons are a crucial input for gamma rhythm generation. Inhibition of PV interneurons attenuates gamma oscillations, whereas driving PV neuronal activity initiates gamma-frequency rhythms [62]. Excitatory pyramidal output in the prefrontal cortex is modulated by inhibitory gamma oscillations, largely driven my PV-interneurons, essentially fine-tuning the circuit and allowing for proper working memory function. Conclusively, PFC-dependent working memory involves a symbiotic balance between excitatory pyramidal output and fast inhibitory activity of PV-interneurons, which shapes and fine-tunes the circuit.

15. Parvalbumin interneuronal hypofunctioning in schizophrenia

Schizophrenia is a debilitating neurodevelopmental disorder in which afflicted individuals suffer from cognitive impairments, working memory deficits being a core feature. Unfortunately, available medications poorly treat cognitive symptoms albeit cognitive performance most strongly determines functional outcomes. Working memory function requires fast and synchronous inhibition of pyramidal neuronal networks within the prefrontal cortex, which is regulated by GABAergic neurotransmission. Because individuals afflicted with schizophrenia display reduced frontal cortical gamma oscillatory power in the DLPFC during a working memory task and cognitive impairments are a core feature, disrupted GABAergic signaling is highly implicated in the pathology of this disorder [57, 62]. Glutamic acid decarboxylase (GAD), the enzyme that synthesizes GABA and PV prefrontal expression is reduced in schizophrenia, further demonstrating a GABA deficit in this neuroanatomical region [57, 62, 77–79].

NMDARs have been demonstrated to be vital throughout neurodevelopment, with NR2A specifically involved in the maturation and maintenance of GABAergic PV interneurons. A previous study showed that NR2A hypofunction leads to reduced GAD67 expression and PV immunoreactivity [59]. It is important to note that the reduction in parvalbumin is not due to density (i.e., interneuronal cell number), but rather a decrease in protein level expression. Researchers hypothesized that this suppressed expression in GAD67, and therefore PV, leads to GABAergic malfunctioning or hypofunctioning [57, 59, 62, 77]. Interestingly, GAD65, the other isoform, does not demonstrate such impairments. Cortical levels of GABA remained unaltered in animals without GAD65, thus demonstrated specificity to the GAD67 isoform [57, 62, 80]. Reductions in GAD67, however, are associated with decreased GAD enzymatic activity as well as GABA levels in the cortex [62, 81]. Individuals suffering from schizophrenia were also reported to have increases in the α_2 subunit of $GABA_A$ receptors and decreased GABA transporter 1 (GAT1) levels. GAT1 are proteins important for the removal of GABA from the synaptic cleft, while the $GABA_A$ α_2 subunit is highly concentrated at the axon initial segment of pyramidal neurons and mediate fast synaptic inhibitory neurotransmission (**Figure 9**). Therefore, this

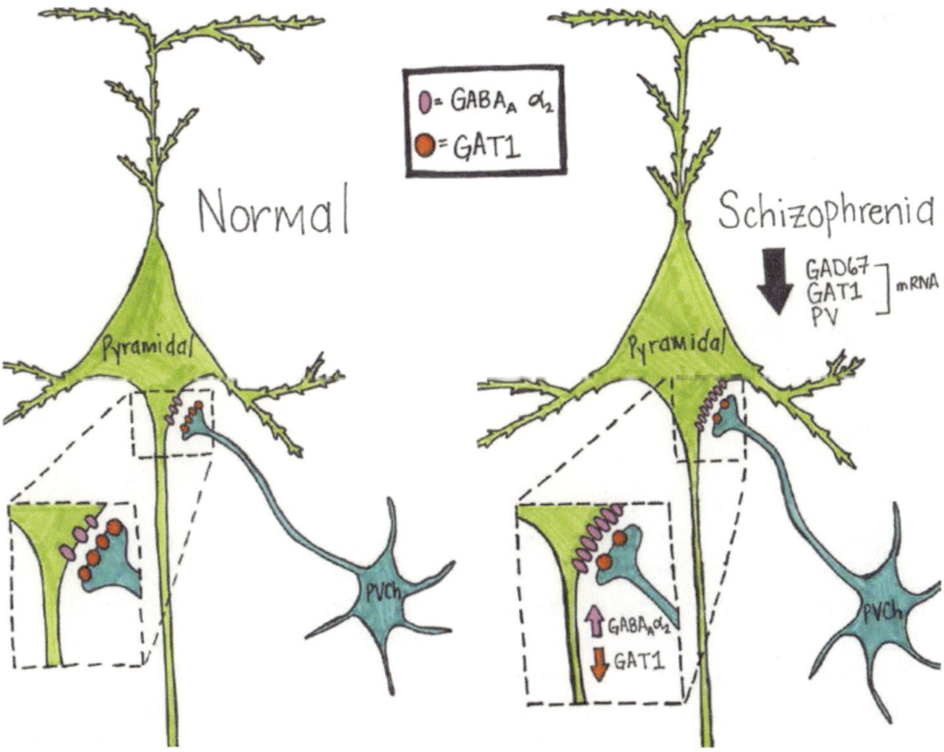

Figure 9. Comparison of normal and schizophrenia synaptic connection at the junction between a parvalbumin chandelier interneuron (PVCh) and a pyramidal axon initial segment. A core feature of schizophrenia is GABergic deficits; in the rebalanced circuitry, presynaptic expression of GABA transporter 1 (GAT1) on the axonal terminals of the GABAergic interneurons is decreased, while the expression of $GABA_A\alpha_2$ receptors at the axon initial segments of pyramidal neurons is increased (Modified from Lewis et al. [62] and Lewis et al. [57]).

inverse correlation is speculated to act as a compensatory mechanism to increase the effect of GABA on postsynaptic cells and return the circuitry back to homeostatic conditions [57, 62, 82].

However, what remains to be unanswered is which proceeds which: NMDA receptor hypofunctioning or GABAergic deficits. In order to understand how cognitive impairments in schizophrenia emerge, we must first uncover the molecular underpinnings that lead to the root of these dysfunctions.

16. Current GABA-targeted therapeutics

In individuals afflicted with schizophrenia, a compensatory mechanism to balance the circuit naturally gets set into motion. In order to offset the shift towards excitation, GAT1 is reduced presynaptically and $GABA_A\alpha_2$ receptors are increased postsynaptically. These changes result in levels of GABA remaining in the synaptic cleft longer and more postsynaptic receptors available for activation. $GABA_A\alpha_2$ receptor agonists offer as a promising therapeutic to pharmacologically target the pathophysiological inhibitory deficit in the DLPFC [62]. $GABA_A\alpha_2$ receptors are predominately located at the axon initial segment of pyramidal neurons and therefore should exhibit limited off-target effects on other domains [83]. $GABA_A\alpha_2$-selective benzodiazepines are a likely candidate because these agents would only activate and potentiate $GABA_A\alpha_2$ receptors in the presence of GABA, preventing dysregulated inhibition that would otherwise result from direct activation of these receptors. Treatment with $GABA_A\alpha 2$-selective benzodiazepines might also offer an additive benefit of reducing anxiety in patients, due to the anxiolytic effects that are mediated by $GABA_A\alpha_2$ receptors [62, 84]. In aims to provide better treatment options, further research is warranted to elucidate the underlying mechanism of GABAergic hypofunctioning, which largely contribute to working memory deficits seen in schizophrenia.

17. Summary

Working memory is a key executive function that guides an organism's response by filtering out important information from the external environment and applying relevant details towards a goal-directed behavior. This process requires the output of a specialized circuit localized within the prefrontal cortical circuits. The synchrony between excitatory pyramidal Delay cells, which produce the necessary persistent neuronal activity, and fast-spiking GABAergic neurotransmission, which in turn shape and fine-tunes the pyramidal cell output, underlies working memory. Both the excitatory and inhibitory components (such as NMDARs and $GABA_A$Rs) are crucial in the maintenance of this delicate process, and dysregulation of either likely serves as a pathophysiological process in schizophrenia. Working memory deficits are a core feature of schizophrenia with NMDA and GABA hypofunctioning highly implicated in the etiology of the disease. Future research is warranted for further deciphering whether NMDA hypofunctioning precedes GABAergic deficits or vice versa.

http://dx.doi.org/10.5772/65870

Acknowledgements

This work was supported by NIH R01MH085666, R21MH110678, and NARSAR Independent Investigator Award 2016 from the Brain and Behavior Research Foundation to W.J. Gao.

Declarations/Competing interest

The authors claim no conflicts of interest.

Author details

Sarah A. Monaco#, Austin A. Coley# and Wen-Jun Gao*

*Address all correspondence to: Wgao@drexelmed.edu

Department of Neurobiology and Anatomy, Drexel University College of Medicine, Philadelphia, PA, USA

# These authors contribute equally

References

[1] Buckley, P.F., et al., Psychiatric comorbidities and schizophrenia. Schizophrenia Bulletin, 2009. **35**(2): p. 383–402.

[2] Glantz, L.A. and D.A. Lewis, Decreased dendritic spine density on prefrontal cortical pyramidal neurons in schizophrenia. Archives of General Psychiatry, 2000. **57**(1): p. 65–73.

[3] Kolluri, N., et al., Lamina-specific reductions in dendritic spine density in the prefrontal cortex of subjects with schizophrenia. American Journal of Psychiatry, 2005. **162**(6): p. 1200–1202.

[4] Selemon, L. and P. Goldman-Rakic, The reduced neuropil hypothesis: A circuit based model of schizophrenia. Biological Psychiatry, 1999. **45**: p. 17–25.

[5] Simpson, E.H., C. Kellendonk, and E. Kandel, A possible role for the striatum in the pathogenesis of the cognitive symptoms of schizophrenia. Neuron, 2010. **65**(5): p. 585–596.

[6] Snyder, M.A., A.E. Adelman, and W.J. Gao, Gestational methylazoxymethanol exposure leads to NMDAR dysfunction in hippocampus during early development and lasting deficits in learning. Neuropsychopharmacology, 2013. **38**(2): p. 328–340.

[7] Lau, C.G. and R.S. Zukin, NMDA receptor trafficking in synaptic plasticity and neuropsychiatric disorders. Nature Reviews Neuroscience, 2007. **8**(6): p. 413–426.

[8] Kristiansen, L.V., et al., Changes in NMDA receptor subunits and interacting PSD proteins in dorsolateral prefrontal and anterior cingulate cortex indicate abnormal regional expression in schizophrenia. Molecular Psychiatry, 2006. **11**(8): p. 737–747, 705.

[9] Clinton, S.M., et al., Altered transcript expression of NMDA receptor-associated post-synaptic proteins in the Thalamus of subjects with schizophrenia. American Journal of Psychiatry, 2003. **160**(6): p. 1100–1109.

[10] Javitt, D.C. and S.R. Zukin, Recent advances in the phencyclidine model of schizophrenia. American Journal of Psychiatry, 1991. **148**(10): p. 1301–1308.

[11] Krystal, J.H., et al., Subanesthetic effects of the noncompetitive NMDA antagonist, ketamine, in humans: Psychotomimetic, perceptual, cognitive, and neuroendocrine responses. Archives of General Psychiatry, 1994. **51**(3): p. 199–214.

[12] Lahti, A.C., et al., Subanesthetic Doses of Ketamine Stimulate Psychosis in Schizophrenia. Neuropsychopharmacology, 1995. **13**(1): p. 9–19.

[13] Stone, J.M., Glutamatergic antipsychotic drugs: a new dawn in the treatment of schizophrenia? Therapeutic Advances in Psychopharmacology, 2011. **1**(1): p. 5–18.

[14] Cioffi, C.L., Modulation of NMDA receptor function as a treatment for schizophrenia. Bioorganic and Medicinal Chemistry Letters, 2013. **23**(18): p. 5034–5044.

[15] Soares, D.C., et al., DISC1: structure, function, and therapeutic potential for major mental illness. ACS Chemical Neuroscience, 2011. **2**(11): p. 609–632.

[16] Porteous, D.J., et al., DISC1 as a genetic risk factor for schizophrenia and related major mental illness: response to Sullivan. Molecular Psychiatry, 2014. **19**(2): p. 141–143.

[17] Tiwari, A.K., et al., Genetics in schizophrenia: where are we and what next? Dialogues in Clinical Neuroscience, 2010. **12**(3): p. 289–303.

[18] Collingridge, G.L., et al., The NMDA receptor as a target for cognitive enhancement. Neuropharmacology, 2013. **64**: p. 13–26.

[19] Dumas, T.C., Developmental regulation of cognitive abilities: modified composition of a molecular switch turns on associative learning. Progress in Neurobiology, 2005. **76**(3): p. 189–211.

[20] Wang, H., et al., A specialized NMDA receptor function in layer 5 recurrent microcircuitry of the adult rat prefrontal cortex. Proceedings of the National Academy of Sciences of the United States of America, 2008. **105**(43): p. 16791–16796.

[21] Monaco, S.A., Y. Gulchina, and W.J. Gao, NR2B subunit in the prefrontal cortex: a double-edged sword for working memory function and psychiatric disorders. Neuroscience and Biobehavioral Reviews, 2015. **56**: p. 127–38.

[22] Amen, D.G., et al., Brain SPECT imaging in complex psychiatric cases: an evidence-based, underutilized tool. The Open Neuroimaging Journal, 2011. **5**: p. 40–48.

[23] Weickert, C.S., et al., Molecular evidence of N-methyl-D-aspartate receptor hypofunction in schizophrenia. Molecular Psychiatry, 2013. **18**(11): p. 1185–1192.

[24] Fromer, M., et al., De novo mutations in schizophrenia implicate synaptic networks. Nature, 2014. **506**(7487): p. 179–184.

[25] Purcell, S.M., et al., A polygenic burden of rare disruptive mutations in schizophrenia. Nature, 2014. **506**(7487): p. 185–190.

[26] Krystal, J.H., A. Anand, and B. Moghaddam, Effects of NMDA receptor antagonists: implications for the pathophysiology of schizophrenia. Archives of General Psychiatry, 2002. **59**(7): p. 663–664.

[27] Meltzer, H.Y., et al., Translating the N-methyl-D-aspartate receptor antagonist model of schizophrenia to treatments for cognitive impairment in schizophrenia. International Journal of Neuropsychopharmacology, 2013. **16**(10): p. 2181–2194.

[28] Taya, S., et al., DISC1 regulates the transport of the NUDEL/LIS1/14-3-3ε complex through Kinesin-1. The Journal of Neuroscience, 2007. **27**(1): p. 15–26.

[29] Shinoda, T., et al., DISC1 regulates neurotrophin-induced axon elongation via interaction with Grb2. The Journal of Neuroscience, 2007. **27**(1): p. 4–14.

[30] Sullivan, P.F., Questions about DISC1 as a genetic risk factor for schizophrenia. Molecular Psychiatry, 2013. **18**(10): p. 1050–1052.

[31] Pletnikov, M.V., et al., Inducible expression of mutant human DISC1 in mice is associated with brain and behavioral abnormalities reminiscent of schizophrenia. Molecular Psychiatry, 2007. **13**(2): p. 173–186.

[32] Cash-Padgett, T. and H. Jaaro-Peled, DISC1 mouse models as a tool to decipher gene-environment interactions in psychiatric disorders. Frontiers in Behavioral Neuroscience, 2013. **7**: p. 113.

[33] Spear, The adolescent brain and age-related behavioral manifestations. Neuroscience and Biobehavioral Reviews, 2000. **24**: p. 417–463.

[34] Snyder, M.A. and W.J. Gao. NMDA hypofunction as a convergence point for progression and symptoms of schizophrenia. Frontiers in Cellular Neuroscience, 2013. **7**: p. 31.

[35] Bibb, J.A., et al., Cognition enhancement strategies. The Journal of Neuroscience, 2010. **30**(45): p. 14987–14992.

[36] Penzes, P., et al., Dendritic spine pathology in neuropsychiatric disorders. Nature Neuroscience, 2011. **14**(3): p. 285–293.

[37] Omkumar, R.V., et al., Identification of a phosphorylation site for calcium/calmodulin-dependent protein kinase II in the NR2B subunit of the N-Methyl-D-aspartate receptor. Journal of Biological Chemistry, 1996. **271**(49): p. 31670–31678.

[38] Raman, I.M., G. Tong, and C.E. Jahr, β-adrenergic regulation of synaptic NMDA receptors by cAMP-dependent protein kinase. Neuron, 1996. **16**(2): p. 415–421.

[39] Li, B.-S., et al., Regulation of NMDA receptors by cyclin-dependent kinase-5. Proceedings of the National Academy of Sciences of the United States of America, 2001. **98**(22): p. 12742–12747.

[40] Chung, H.J., et al., Regulation of the NMDA receptor complex and trafficking by activity-dependent phosphorylation of the NR2B subunit PDZ ligand. The Journal of Neuroscience, 2004. **24**(45): p. 10248–10259.

[41] Hradetzky, E., et al., The methylazoxymethanol acetate (MAM-E17) rat model: molecular and functional effects in the hippocampus. Neuropsychopharmacology, 2012. **37**(2): p. 364–377.

[42] Jaaro-Peled, H., et al., Neurodevelopmental mechanisms of schizophrenia: understanding disturbed postnatal brain maturation through neuregulin-1-ErbB4 and DISC1. Trends in Neurosciences, 2009. **32**(9): p. 485–495.

[43] Sanna, P.P., et al., Phosphatidylinositol 3-kinase is required for the expression but not for the induction or the maintenance of long-term potentiation in the hippocampal CA1 region. The Journal of Neuroscience, 2002. **22**(9): p. 3359–3365.

[44] Balu, D.T., et al., Akt1 deficiency in schizophrenia and impairment of hippocampal plasticity and function. Hippocampus, 2012. **22**(2): p. 230–240.

[45] Mills, C.N., et al., Emerging roles of glycogen synthase kinase 3 in the treatment of brain tumors. Frontiers in Molecular Neuroscience, 2011. **4**: p. 47.

[46] Chen, P., et al., Glycogen synthase kinase 3 regulates N-Methyl-d-aspartate receptor channel trafficking and function in cortical neurons. Molecular Pharmacology, 2007. **72**(1): p. 40–51.

[47] Hashimoto, R., et al., Impact of the DISC1 Ser704Cys polymorphism on risk for major depression, brain morphology and ERK signaling. Human Molecular Genetics, 2006. **15**(20): p. 3024–3033.

[48] Lipina, T.V., et al., Synergistic interactions between PDE4B and GSK-3: DISC1 mutant mice. Neuropharmacology, 2012. **62**(3): p. 1252–1562.

[49] Lipina, T.V., et al., Genetic and pharmacological evidence for schizophrenia-related disc1 interaction with GSK-3. Synapse (New York, N.Y.), 2011. **65**(3): p. 234–248.

[50] Gilmartin, M.R., J.L. Kwapis, and F.J. Helmstetter, NR2A- and NR2B-containing NMDA receptors in the prelimbic medial prefrontal cortex differentially mediate trace, delay, and contextual fear conditioning. Learning and Memory, 2013. **20**(6): p. 290–294.

[51] Wang, X.J., Synaptic reverberation underlying mnemonic persistent activity. Trends in Neurosciences, 2001. **24**(8): p. 455–463.

[52] Tsukada, H., et al., Chronic NMDA antagonism impairs working memory, decreases extracellular dopamine, and increases D1 receptor binding in prefrontal cortex of conscious monkeys. Neuropsychopharmacology, 2005. **30**(10): p. 1861–1869.

[53] Hetem, L.A., et al., Effect of a subanesthetic dose of ketamine on memory and conscious awareness in healthy volunteers. Psychopharmacology (Berl), 2000. **152**(3): p. 283–288.

[54] Malhotra, A.K., et al., NMDA receptor function and human cognition: the effects of ketamine in healthy volunteers. Neuropsychopharmacology, 1996. **14**(5): p. 301–307.

[55] Newcomer, J.W., et al., Ketamine-induced NMDA receptor hypofunction as a model of memory impairment and psychosis. Neuropsychopharmacology, 1999. **20**(2): p. 106–118.

[56] Parwani, A., et al., The effects of a subanesthetic dose of ketamine on verbal memory in normal volunteers. Psychopharmacology (Berl), 2005. **183**(3): p. 265–274.

[57] Lewis, D.A., et al., Cortical parvalbumin interneurons and cognitive dysfunction in schizophrenia. Trends in Neurosciences, 2012. **35**(1): p. 57–67.

[58] Zhang, Z. and Q.Q. Sun, Development of NMDA NR2 subunits and their roles in critical period maturation of neocortical GABAergic interneurons. Developmental Neurobiology, 2011. **71**(3): p. 221–245.

[59] Kinney, J.W., et al., A specific role for NR2A-containing NMDA receptors in the maintenance of parvalbumin and GAD67 immunoreactivity in cultured interneurons. The Journal of Neuroscience, 2006. **26**(5): p. 1604–1615.

[60] Wonders, C.P. and S.A. Anderson, The origin and specification of cortical interneurons. Nature Reviews Neuroscience, 2006. **7**(9): p. 687–696.

[61] Markram, H., et al., Interneurons of the neocortical inhibitory system. Nature Reviews Neuroscience, 2004. **5**(10): p. 793–807.

[62] Lewis, D.A., T. Hashimoto, and D.W. Volk, Cortical inhibitory neurons and schizophrenia. Nature Reviews Neuroscience, 2005. **6**(4): p. 312–324.

[63] Bettler, B., et al., Molecular structure and physiological functions of GABA(B) receptors. Physiological Reviews, 2004. **84**(3): p. 835–867.

[64] Emson, P.C., GABA(B) receptors: structure and function. Progress in Brain Research, 2007. **160**: p. 43–57.

[65] Jacob, T.C., S.J. Moss, and R. Jurd, GABA(A) receptor trafficking and its role in the dynamic modulation of neuronal inhibition. Nature Reviews Neuroscience, 2008. **9**(5): p. 331–343.

[66] Laurie, D.J., W. Wisden, and P.H. Seeburg, The distribution of thirteen GABAA receptor subunit mRNAs in the rat brain. III. Embryonic and postnatal development. The Journal of Neuroscience, 1992. **12**(11): p. 4151–4172.

[67] Nutt, D., GABAA receptors: subtypes, regional distribution, and function. Journal of Clinical Sleep Medicine, 2006. **2**(2): p. S7–S11.

[68] Sigel, E. and M.E. Steinmann, Structure, function, and modulation of GABA(A) receptors. The Journal of Biological Chemistry, 2012. **287**(48): p. 40224–40231.

[69] Vithlani, M., M. Terunuma, and S.J. Moss, The dynamic modulation of GABA(A) receptor trafficking and its role in regulating the plasticity of inhibitory synapses. Physiological Reviews, 2011. **91**(3): p. 1009–1022.

[70] Chebib, M. and G.A. Johnston, The 'ABC' of GABA receptors: a brief review. Clinical and Experimental Pharmacology Physiology, 1999. **26**(11): p. 937–940.

[71] Goldman-Rakic, P.S., Regional and cellular fractionation of working memory. Proceedings of the National Academy of Sciences of the United States of America, 1996. **93**(24): p. 13473–13480.

[72] Baddeley, A., Working memory. Science, 1992. **255**(5044): p. 556–559.

[73] Fuster, J.M. and G.E. Alexander, Neuron activity related to short-term memory. Science, 1971. **173**(3997): p. 652–654.

[74] Goldman-Rakic, P.S., Cellular basis of working memory. Neuron, 1995. **14**(3): p. 477–485.

[75] Sawaguchi, T., M. Matsumura, and K. Kubota, Delayed response deficits produced by local injection of bicuculline into the dorsolateral prefrontal cortex in Japanese macaque monkeys. Experimental Brain Research, 1989. **75**(3): p. 457–469.

[76] Howard, M.W., et al., Gamma oscillations correlate with working memory load in humans. Cerebral Cortex, 2003. **13**(12): p. 1369–1374.

[77] Akbarian, S., et al., Gene expression for glutamic acid decarboxylase is reduced without loss of neurons in prefrontal cortex of schizophrenics. Archives of General Psychiatry, 1995. **52**(4): p. 258–266.

[78] Guidotti, A., et al., Decrease in reelin and glutamic acid decarboxylase67 (GAD67) expression in schizophrenia and bipolar disorder: a postmortem brain study. Archives of General Psychiatry, 2000. **57**(11): p. 1061–1069.

[79] Volk, D.W., et al., Decreased glutamic acid decarboxylase67 messenger RNA expression in a subset of prefrontal cortical gamma-aminobutyric acid neurons in subjects with schizophrenia. Archives of General Psychiatry, 2000. **57**(3): p. 237–245.

[80] Asada, H., et al., Mice lacking the 65 kDa isoform of glutamic acid decarboxylase (GAD65) maintain normal levels of GAD67 and GABA in their brains but are susceptible to seizures. Biochemical and Biophysical Research Communications, 1996. **229**(3): p. 891–895.

[81] Asada, H., et al., Cleft palate and decreased brain gamma-aminobutyric acid in mice lacking the 67-kDa isoform of glutamic acid decarboxylase. Proceedings of the National Academy of Sciences of the United States of America, 1997. **94**(12): p. 6496–9.

http://dx.doi.org/10.5772/65870

[82] Volk, D.W., et al., Reciprocal alterations in pre- and postsynaptic inhibitory markers at chandelier cell inputs to pyramidal neurons in schizophrenia. Cerebral Cortex, 2002. **12**(10): p. 1063–70.

[83] Nusser, Z., et al., Differential synaptic localization of two major gamma-aminobutyric acid type A receptor alpha subunits on hippocampal pyramidal cells. Proceedings of the National Academy of Sciences of the United States of America, 1996. **93**(21): p. 11939–11944.

[84] Low, K., et al., Molecular and neuronal substrate for the selective attenuation of anxiety. Science, 2000. **290**(5489): p. 131–134.

Chapter 2

Changes in DNA Sequence and Methylation Contribute to the Predisposition of Schizophrenia: Toward an Epigenetic Therapy

Melkaye G. Melka, Christina A. Castellani and Shiva M. Singh

Additional information is available at the end of the chapter

http://dx.doi.org/10.5772/65905

Abstract

Schizophrenia has a heterogeneous and complex etiology that includes multiple candidate genes affected by a variety of mutational mechanisms including epigenetics, functional pathways, and environmental factors. This chapter mainly focuses on reviewing two sets of studies. The first one is whole-genome next-generation sequencing datasets involving monozygotic twins discordant for schizophrenia. The findings suggest that *de novo* sequence variations may underlie the discordance of monozygotic twins for schizophrenia. Second, whole-genome DNA methylation study suggesting the role of DNA methylation in the mechanisms of actions of antipsychotic drugs in treating the disorder as well as the manifestation of side effects such as metabolic disorders. Furthermore, we are reporting original research results using next-generation mitochondrial DNA sequence analysis of a pair of monozygotic twins discordant for schizophrenia as well as their mother. The chapter sheds light on the interplay between sequence variations and epigenetic signatures, including DNA methylation changes, in the etiology and pathophysiology of schizophrenia. Given the dynamic nature of methylation, it may be possible to develop a new treatment strategy for schizophrenia that is based on reversion of genomic methylation. This may involve environmental, dietary, and/or pharmaceutical approaches.

Keywords: schizophrenia, twins, sequence variation, DNA methylation

1. Introduction

The treatment of schizophrenia involves the suppression of hallucinations, delusions, agitation, and an array of behavioral problems that often accompany these symptoms [1]. When acute symptoms start to subside with antipsychotic drug treatment, psychotherapy and rehabilitation interventions can be undertaken. The heterogeneity of schizophrenia may account for concentration of the disease in some families, reduced concordance between monozygotic twins, and patient-specific causations. The identity of genes and pathways involved in schizophrenia and the mechanisms affecting them are forthcoming. This development has identified important insights including the fact that a relatively large number of genes affected in schizophrenia belong to relatively few critical pathways. This includes the Dopamine pathway that has provided the foundation for the development of primary treatment of the disease. There is an opportunity to focus on additional affected pathways for the treatment of a subset of patients. One of the mechanisms that may affect schizophrenia-related pathways is DNA methylation. This chapter will discuss primary molecular studies that support a threshold model for this complex disease, including complete genome sequences of monozygotic twins discordant (MZD). Specifically, we identify patient-specific genes that may be affected by a variety of mutational mechanisms, including DNA methylation. Here, the predisposition for the disease is realized on a threshold scale (**Figure 1**) via mutations involving a variety of mechanisms including sequence variations and copy number variations in nuclear genes as well as changes in genome-wide DNA methylation [2, 3]. The threshold model can only be tested on monozygotic twins discordant for the disease. Next, we will argue for the direct role of DNA methylation in schizophrenia using two sets of independent results; methylation differences between MZD twins and tissue-specific response of olanzapine (antipsychotic) treatment in rats *in vivo* [4, 5].

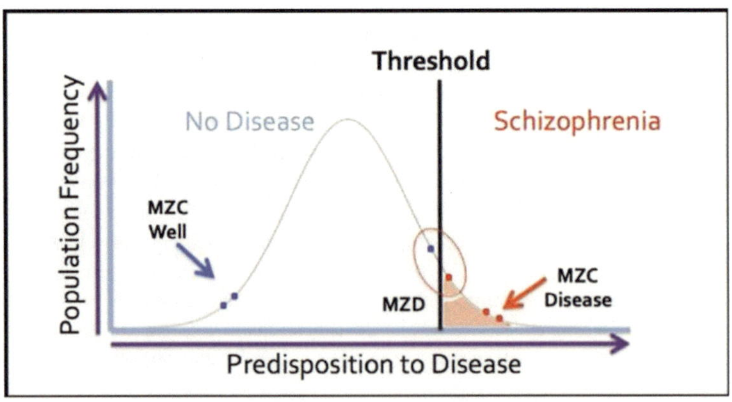

Figure 1. A threshold model for predisposition to schizophrenia in monozygotic twins discordant (MZD) for schizophrenia [2].

We will also discuss three facets of schizophrenia and their implications in the development of any strategy for amelioration: (i) the role of *de novo* sequence variations (nuclear and mtDNA) in the etiology and treatment of psychiatric disorders, including schizophrenia; (ii) the involvement of DNA methylation in the development of psychiatric disorders, particularly schizophrenia; and (iii) the interplay between DNA sequence variation and DNA methylation. The insights covered will be incorporated into the development of strategies toward personalized medicine for the treatment of psychiatric disorders.

2. Role of sequence variations in the etiology and treatment of psychosis

A growing body of evidence suggests the significance of genetic variants in the etiology of mental health disorders, including schizophrenia. For example, the Psychiatric Genomics Consortium identified several SNPs that are associated with major psychiatric disorders including schizophrenia [6], which included *CACNA1C* variants that have been previously associated with autism [7]. Also, angiotensin-converting enzyme (ACE) gene insertion/deletion polymorphism was reported to be associated with schizophrenia susceptibility as well as the severity of schizophrenia depressive symptoms in a Chinese population [8]. According to the schizophrenia-working group of the Psychiatric Genetic Consortium, the expression of the C4 gene was affected by SNPs in the gene resulting in putative synapse elimination in schizophrenia patients [9]. It has recently been reported that 15 of 48 schizophrenia cases were found to carry rare or novel missense coding variants in four signaling genes studied. These findings suggest that single genes harboring *de novo* mutations in individuals with psychosis as compared to healthy controls may play a critical role in influencing the phenotypes of psychosis and hence may be potential targets for developing treatment strategies. A study from our lab reported that copy number variants (CNVs) in monozygotic twins discordant for schizophrenia could be an important underlying factor in the discordance of the twins for the disease [3]. The findings identified several CNVs and genes, in four of the six twin pairs studied, that were previously implicated in mental health disorders. These findings suggest a role for CNVs in the discordance of twins for schizophrenia.

Similarly, unpublished studies from our lab on complete genomes of two pairs of monozygotic twins discordant for schizophrenia showed multiple individual sequence-specific differences between cotwins. The observed differences included small nucleotide changes (single nucleotide variation, block substitutions, and small indels), copy number variations, and structural variations that were unique to either the affected or healthy cotwins. Also, by comparing the sequence differences between cotwins with that of their parents, it was possible to identify *de novo* variants. The study revealed several genes and gene-networks that may have predisposed the affected cotwins to the disease corroborating the fact that *de novo* variations between cotwins may be an underlying factor for their discordance to the disease.

Due to the fact that there has been no single gene identified that is responsible for causing the disorder, it is imperative that future research be focused on the polygenetic nature of schizophrenia, as well as the networks and pathways relevant to neurodevelopment and function. A recent study identified genes and pathways associated with psychosis in 22q11.2 deletion syndrome subjects [10]. The study revealed specific pathways affected in 22q11 deletion

Syndrome carriers with psychosis and autistic spectrum disorders. Expression changes associated with psychosis symptoms in 22q11 deletion syndrome was also associated with pathways involved in transcriptional regulation. In addition, schizophrenia was reported to be the only psychiatric disorder observed at a higher rate in 22q11 deletion syndrome compared to other neurodevelopmental disorders [11, 12].

The 22q11.2 deletion represents one of the most established genetic risk factors for the development of psychiatric disorders. Our lab also reported the effect of DNA methylation in the promoter regions of genes located in the microdeletion region on chromosome 22. Accordingly, from a set of genes located in the 22q11.2 microdeletion region that has been previously implicated in psychosis, 29 genes showed increased DNA methylation in their promoters, following olanzapine treatment [13]. In that study, the effect of the antipsychotic drug was revealed through significantly increased ($p < 0.01$) DNA methylation of genes affecting several networks including neurological disease, inflammatory disease, inflammatory response, cancer, tumor morphology, and cell death and survival.

An increased number of studies suggest that rare genetic variations play an important role in the genetic etiology of schizophrenia. However, the existence of rare genetic variations may not always lead to the predisposition of schizophrenia. For example, a rare missense variation in *UCL13B* was identified by whole-exome sequencing, which was present in five of six schizophrenia-affected individuals but not in eight unaffected individuals [14]. In a follow-up case-control study of two independent Japanese populations, there was no significant association between this missense variation and schizophrenia [14].

Chr	Position	Reference allele	Sample allele	Variation type	Gene regions	Gene symbol	Sample call quality	Sample read depth in G/H/F	Translation impact
M	8701	A	G	SNV	Exonic	MT-ATP6	255	600/680/611	Missense
M	8860	A	G	SNV	Exonic	MT-ATP6	255	336/367/322	Missense
M	10819	A	G	SNV	Exonic	MT-ND4	255	729/714/667	Synonymous
M	10873	T	C	SNV	Exonic	MT-ND4	255	613/662/573	Synonymous
M	11719	G	A	SNV	Exonic	MT-ND4	255	544/652/562	Synonymous

Note: G/H/F: stands for healthy cotwin, affected cotwin, and their mom, respectively; Chr: chromosome.

Table 1. Mitochondrial single nucleotide variations detected in the discordant twins as well as their mother.

In addition to our analysis of nuclear DNA sequence variation, we have also conducted mitochondrial DNA sequence analysis involving a pair of monozygotic twins discordant for schizophrenia and their mother. Ingenuity Variant Analysis (Ingenuity System Inc, CA, USA) identified no difference in the sequence variations between the discordant twins as well as their mother. All of the biologically relevant variations detected were single nucleotide variations (SNVs) in exonic regions of the *MT-ATP6* and *MT-ND4* genes (**Table 1**). The translational

http://dx.doi.org/10.5772/65905

impact of the variation found in *MT-ATP6* was predicted to be *missense* while that of *MT-ND4* was predicted to be *synonymous*. All of the single nucleotide variations found in the mitochondria were detected in both of the twins and their mother. As we will discuss in the subsequent sections, despite the identification of these biologically relevant sequence variations in all samples, their interaction with epigenetic signatures including DNA methylation may differ between individuals and lead to differences in susceptibility to disease.

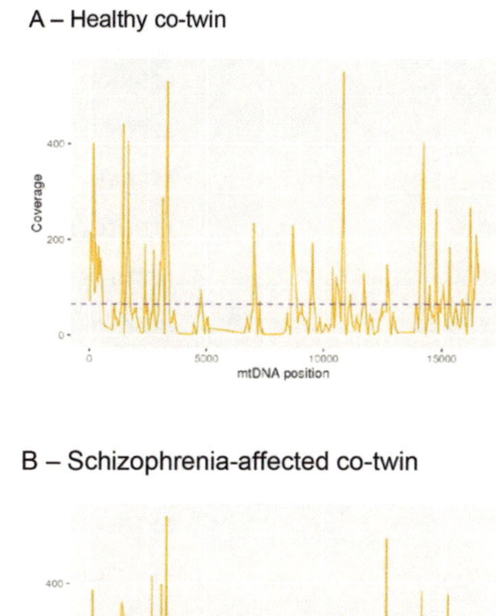

Figure 2. The dotted line in purple shows the mean sequencing coverage of the mitochondrial genome for each sample. (A) Healthy cotwin. (B) Schizophrenia-affected cotwin. (C) Mother of the twins.

Position	Mutation	Locus
10398	A>G	MT-ND3
10819	A>G	MT-ND4
10873	T>C	MT-ND4
11719	G>A	MT-ND4
12705	C>T	MT-ND5
14212	T>C	MT-CYB
1438	A>G	MT-RNR1
14766	C>T	MT-CYB
14905	G>A	MT-CYB
150	C>T	MT-DLOOP2
152	T>C	MT-DLOOP2
15301	G>A	MT-CYB
15326	A>G	MT-CYB
16172	T>C	MT-DLOOP1
16183	A>C	MT-DLOOP1
16189	T>C	MT-DLOOP1
16223	C>T	MT-DLOOP1
1647	T>C	MT-TV
16519	T>C	MT-DLOOP1
195	T>C	MT-DLOOP2
2352	T>C	MT-RNR2
263	A>G	MT-DLOOP2
2706	A>G	MT-RNR2
3316	G>A	MT-ND1
4769	A>G	MT-ND2
7028	C>T	MT-C01
73	A>G	MT-DLOOP2
750	A>G	MT-RNR1
8701	A>G	MT-ATP6
8860	A>G	MT-ATP6
9540	T>C	MT-C03

Table 2. Homoplasmies detected in the discordant twins and their mother.

We used mtDNA-server [15] to identify heteroplasmies. All sites with a log likelihood ratio (LLR) of ≥5 were considered as heteroplasmic sites. This analysis did not identify any heteroplasmies in our samples. Among other reasons, the sequencing coverage may have affected our ability to detect heteroplasmies in the present samples (**Figure 2**). Coverage of ≥10× fold per strand is required on both the forward and reverse strand to accurately identify heteroplasmic sites [15]. We believe that better coverage would more accurately identify heteroplasmies that may have a role in the etiology of schizophrenia. Furthermore, analyzing larger samples may help investigate heteroplasmies and their association with schizophrenia; as it is possible that each patient could signify a specific etiology and pathophysiological manifestation of the disease via his/her unique genetic makeup and epigenomic signature. In another study, novel and rare nonsynonymous mutations were identified in mtDNA genes (*ND6*, *ATP6*, *CYTB*, and *ND2*) in subjects with psychiatric disorders [16]. The authors also reported mtDNA heteroplasmy at a locus that was known to be associated with schizophrenia (*T16519C*). The homoplasmies detected in the aforementioned sample of a pair of twins discordant for schizophrenia and their mother are presented in **Table 2**.

3. The role of DNA methylation in the development of psychosis

DNA methylation represents a core epigenetic mechanism that involves the covalent binding of a methyl group to the 5-carbon position of cytosine, often leading to altered gene expression [17]. DNA methylation is influenced by stochastic events, including exposure to a variety of environmental factors, such as drug treatment [18, 19]. Epigenetic mechanisms, including DNA methylation, regulate normal cognition, neurodevelopment, and function. In addition, DNA sequence variations only explain a small proportion of the heritability of the disease. The remaining heritability, often referred to as missing heritability, could be, at least partially, explained by epigenetic changes. Interestingly, a number of animal model studies of neurodevelopmental disorders signified that reversing the underlying molecular deficits could lead to substantial improvements in function giving hope to effective treatments even starting in adulthood [20]. These points highlight the need to further investigate the role of epigenetic signatures in the etiology and treatment of psychiatric disorders, including schizophrenia.

With this in mind, our lab has performed two sets of studies on DNA methylation in schizophrenia. The first study focused on two pairs of monozygotic twins discordant for schizophrenia and their parents to investigate differences in genome-wide DNA methylation using a NimbleGen Methylation Promoter Microarray. Since monozygotic twins share nearly identical DNA, the study represents an ideal design to investigate the role of DNA methylation in the etiology of the disease. The genomic DNA was processed at ArrayStar (Rockville, MD, USA). Pair files were analyzed with the tiling workflow in Partek Genomics Suite version 6.6 (St. Louis, Missouri, USA). Details of the methodology have been previously described [4]. As a result, differentially methylated regions (DMRs) were identified between discordant monozygotic twins. Some of the DMRs were shared with parents of the discordant twins while others represented *de novo* methylation changes [4]. The study also reported that 27 genes were affected by DMR changes that were commonly detected in the schizophrenia-affected member of the two discordant monozygotic pairs of unrelated families. Many of these genes were found to be a part of the histone coding gene family, which has been previously linked to the causation of schizophrenia [21–23]. Moreover, the identified genes affected by DMRs were linked to specific networks including "cell death and survival" and "cellular movement and immune cell trafficking" [4]. Interestingly, those genes and their networks have been previously associated with the etiology of schizophrenia. The findings of this particular study corroborated the notion that DNA methylation may play a critical role in the discordance of monozygotic twins for schizophrenia. The results also shed light on the relevance of gene-specific DNA methylation changes and on the involvement of multiple genes harboring methylation changes across specific pathways in the discordance of monozygotic twins for schizophrenia.

The second study comprised an animal model experiment investigating genome-wide DNA methylation changes following the administration of a therapeutic dose of olanzapine in rats *in vivo*. Hippocampus and cerebellum brain regions were used and liver was included as a nonbrain tissue [5]. As a result, our study revealed that DNA methylation is not only involved in the etiology of mental health disorders, but also may be the underlying mechanism by which antipsychotic drugs function in treating the disorder. This was supported by a number of pathways significantly influenced by methylation changes. These included "nervous system development and function, tissue morphology, cellular assembly and organization," (**Figure 3**). These findings suggested that an increase or decrease in DNA methylation of specific gene promoters, following olanzapine treatment, might decrease or increase transcriptional efficiency [37, 38], specifically in the hippocampus. The hippocampus is viewed as one of the primary sites associated with psychotic symptoms [7, 24, 25]. We also reported that the *dopamine-DARPP32 feedback in cAMP signaling* pathway ($p < 1.6E\text{-}3$) was the most significant pathway identified in the hippocampus region of the olanzapine-treated rat brain. Neurons in the midbrain release dopamine, which modulates *cAmp* (cyclic adenosine 3,5-monophosphate) production by activating dopamine receptors [1]. These results may suggest that antipsychotic effects of olanzapine involve alterations in gene-specific methylation that would lead to disregulation of genes involved in the dopamine *DARPP32 feedback in cAmp signaling* pathway. This includes several differentially methylated genes such as *Drd1/5* and *Nos1*. It is an established fact that dopamine blockade leads to the progressive treatment of psychosis while its disturbance leads to the manifestation of psychosis [26]. And, all currently used antipsychotics block postsynaptic D2 receptors [27].

Schizophrenia patients either partially respond to antipsychotic drugs or do not respond at all [28]. This may be due to several factors, and one possibility is the delay in the onset of therapeutic actions partly or fully influenced by downstream effects, such as altered transcription [29, 30]. As such, differentially methylated genes involved in the dopamine-signaling pathway may stop or reduce transcription and gene expression [17, 29, 30].

Significant hypomethylation in two CpG sites of the *FAM63B* gene in bipolar disorder patients have been recently reported [31]. Their findings plus previous hypomethylation results reported in another study involving schizophrenia patients suggest that *FAM63B* may be a common risk gene for both disorders. Although the authors reported correlation in methylation levels at the two sites, they did not find significant association of DNA methylation with

http://dx.doi.org/10.5772/65905

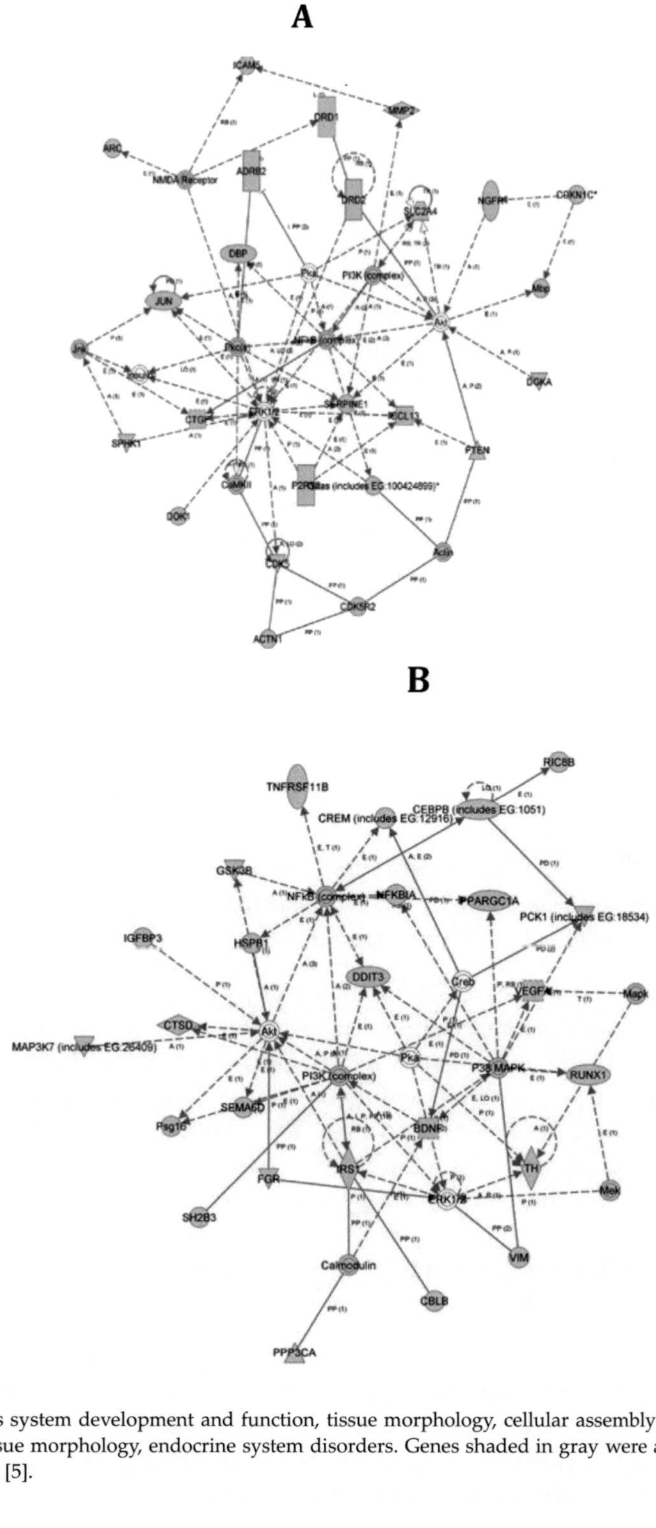

Figure 3. (A) Nervous system development and function, tissue morphology, cellular assembly and organization. (B) Metabolic disease, tissue morphology, endocrine system disorders. Genes shaded in gray were affected by changes in promoter methylation [5].

nearby SNPs, which may further corroborate the biological significance of identifying epigenetic signatures in addition to conducting genome-wide association analyses. On their own, association analyses will not always reveal risk variants or genes due to their limitations such as low statistical power or the presence of genotyping error as well as the detection of false positives.

Different brain regions as well as a variety of cell types are known to have different epigenetic signatures, and depending on the subpopulations analyzed, specific cell types may even show different epigenetic signatures within their own subpopulation [32, 33]. These reported differences in epigenetic signatures of different brain regions and our observations of significant differences in DNA methylation patterns of hippocampus and cerebellum in a rat model study, reflect the possibility that these epigenetic signatures may play a role in regulating gene expression and thereby causing psychiatric disorders including schizophrenia.

Several CpGs have been reported to show significant differences in DNA methylation levels in psychosis cases [34]. These results shed light on the significance of epigenetic signatures in the causes and treatment of mental health disorders. Our previous studies revealed brain tissue-specific DNA methylation changes [5]. As a result, scientists are now advising for caution when interpreting the findings of DNA methylation differences in schizophrenia affected and healthy subjects using peripheral tissues, including blood samples [35].

As we noted in our previous reports, olanzapine caused an increase or a decrease in methylation of genes previously implicated in schizophrenia, which may reflect the fact that olanzapine could result in the recovery of psychiatric symptoms via mechanisms involving DNA methylation. Among the genes that showed a decrease in methylation in hippocampus is *Map6*, which is implicated in schizophrenia [36], and involved in molecular transport, nervous system development, and function [5]. This implies that methylation may serve an intermediary role whose actual effect is realized through gene expression.

Apart from the involvement of DNA methylation in the treatment of schizophrenia via antipsychotic administration, methylation changes may also affect genes and pathways that reflect the side effects of the drugs. In a genome-wide assessment, our studies showed methylation changes in several genes and pathways that may alter metabolomics leading to the efficacy as well as side effects of olanzapine. The side effects were reflected by significant increases in body weight gain and a pathway affecting metabolic disorders. Interestingly, genetic variations in various genes including *BDNF* have been implicated in antipsychotic-induced weight gain [37]. However, the relationship between sequence variations and methylation changes in leading to the predisposition of individuals to the disease, their role in the efficacy of antipsychotic treatment, and also their role in the side effects of the drugs remains to be investigated.

It is an established fact that genomic imprinting is an epigenetic phenomenon by which certain genes are expressed in a parent-of-origin specific manner [38]. Also, X-chromosome inactivation invariably involves epigenetic phenomenon [39, 40]. The genomic distributions of epimutations play an important role in their effects on the disorder. In particular, we would like to emphasize that not all observed epigenetic changes in the genome play a role in the regulation of gene expression. Although most epimutations located in nonpromoter regions do not often lead to changes in gene expression, epigenetic signatures in the promoter regions are often associated with regulation of gene expressions [29, 41]. Interestingly, long-lasting alterations in DNA methylation and their effect on neurodevelopmental disorders have been reported [42]. However, changes in DNA methylation needs to be interpreted with caution, as methylation and its function are context-dependent [43]. More importantly, effects of epimutations on neurodevelopmental disorders are tissue-specific, cell-type, and organ specific [44, 45]. Interestingly, our lab reported tissue-specific changes in promoter DNA methylation of several psychosis related genes using hippocampus, cerebellum, and liver samples [5].

Overall, the results from our lab and elsewhere suggest that aberrant DNA methylation in a set of candidate genes may be involved in mental disorders, including schizophrenia [46]. Also, it may explain the therapeutic efficacy, side effects, and individual specificity of responses to antipsychotic treatments. They may result from changes in tissue-specific DNA methylation in a set of genes [5, 13, 47, 48]. However, DNA methylation changes in mental health patients and their effects on the expression of psychosis relevant genes as well as the development of psychotic symptoms require attention in future studies. Also, effects of DNA methylation on the expression of specific sets of genes leading to the development of schizophrenia, requires further investigation. To this effect, the use of endophenotypes (intermediate phenotypes that are quantifiable traits of the disease) may help facilitate the investigation of the underlying biological basis of schizophrenia. The United States Food and Drug Administration has accepted endophenotypes as therapeutic treatment targets [49]. Further, our study based on two sets of studies (a rat model investigating effects of olanzapine on DNA methylation of brain regions, and monozygotic twins discordant for schizophrenia) revealed genes and gene networks commonly affected in the two sets of studies. The findings reflect the fact that a considerable portion of the observed methylation changes are likely to be caused by antipsychotic drugs in both studies [50]. Also, it is likely that some of the methylation changes seen can be attributed to the underlying factors that predispose patients to the disorder. Further studies are still needed to confirm the role of methylation changes in the etiology and pathophysiology of the disease.

4. Interplay between DNA sequence variation and DNA methylation

The role of DNA methylation in gene regulation and the interplay between genomic sequence variations and various environmental features as well as their implications on disease phenotypes remains to be investigated. However, studies support the role of DNA methylation in regulatory interactions influencing gene expression [51]. It is also established that there is an interplay between sequence variation, DNA methylation, and gene expression [52]. A recent study has highlighted the fact that mutated CpG sites (CpG-SNPs) could play a critical role in the cause and treatment of the disease [34].

Our lab recently identified several genes that differ between the affected and unaffected members of two monozygotic twin pairs discordant for schizophrenia. The differences were assessed using a genome-wide methylation promoter array and complete genome sequences. The results shed light on a number of facts. First, monozygotic twins differ in both DNA methylation as well as *de novo* sequence variations. Antipsychotic drugs could have caused the observed DNA methylation changes as was evidenced in our rat model study discussed above. Also, there is a possibility that DNA methylation changes could be caused by *de novo* events. It has been reported that differences in genetic components underlie the differences in DNA methylation profiles observed between individuals [53]. Second, some genes that were affected by differential promoter methylation between discordant monozygotic twins also harbor a number of different types of sequence variations [2]. Some of the variations may represent *de novo* sequence variations. Third, a number of the observed changes are located in known candidate genes for schizophrenia. Thus, the genes harboring promoter DNA methylation changes could contribute to neuropsychiatric disorders, including schizophrenia. Moreover, when the DNA sequence differences were analyzed independently, additional previously reported candidate genes of schizophrenia were identified (unpublished data) suggesting that these findings may reflect that many of the previously identified candidate genes of schizophrenia can be revealed by differences in DNA sequence. These findings also highlight the patient-specific nature of these differences. Any sequence variation or promoter DNA methylation between a patient and their healthy cotwin was considered as a potential predisposing factor for the disease. Overall, the findings to date argue that it is not only sequence variation but also their interactions with chromatin structure and other epigenetic signatures which regulate disease outcomes. Therefore, future studies need to focus on investigating the interactions of sequence variation, including nuclear and mitochondrial DNA sequence variations, with epigenetic signatures, in subjects with psychosis and healthy controls.

Studies in the past support the notion that DNA methylation may play a critical role in the therapeutic efficacy of olanzapine. For example, findings suggest that DNA methylation changes in the promoter regions of several genes including genes located in the 22q11.2 microdeletion region and the cadherin/protocadherin genes impact the response of olanzapine treatment [47]. These impacts have been revealed through the identified pathways that have been previously implicated in psychosis.

In conclusion, the results from our lab and elsewhere corroborated the fact that various types of *de novo* sequence, including copy number variants and their interactions with epigenetic signatures, may underlie the etiology of schizophrenia and also may hold the key to discovery of drug targets in developing personalized medicine for psychosis. Epigenetic changes, DNA methylation in particular, may play a critical role in the therapeutic efficacy of antipsychotic drugs. Overall, the known functions of genes affected by olanzapine-induced DNA methylation changes suggest that DNA methylation differences may underlie the amelioration of psychosis symptoms as well as account for certain adverse effects of drugs used to treat the disorder.

Author details

Melkaye G. Melka, Christina A. Castellani and Shiva M. Singh*

*Address all correspondence to: ssingh@uwo.ca

Department of Biology, University of Western Ontario, London, ON, Canada

References

[1] Svenningsson P, Nishi A, Fisone G, Girault J-A, Nairn AC, Greengard P. DARPP-32: an integrator of neurotransmission. *Annu Rev Pharmacol Toxicol*. 2004;44:269–296. doi: 10.1146/annurev.pharmtox.44.101802.121415.

[2] Castellani CA, Melka MG, Gui JL, O'Reilly RL, Singh SM. Integration of DNA sequence and DNA methylation changes in monozygotic twin pairs discordant for schizophrenia. *Schizophrenia Research*. 2015;169(1–3):433–40.

[3] Castellani CA, Awamleh Z, Melka MG, O'Reilly RL, Singh SM. Copy number variation distribution in six monozygotic twin pairs discordant for schizophrenia. *Twin Res Hum Genet*. 2014;17(2):108–120. doi:10.1017/thg.2014.6.

[4] Castellani CA, Laufer BI, Melka MG, Diehl EJ, O'Reilly RL, Singh SM. DNA methylation differences in monozygotic twin pairs discordant for schizophrenia identifies psychosis related genes and networks. *BMC Med Genomics*. 2015;8(1):17. doi:10.1186/s12920-015-0093-1.

[5] Melka MG, Laufer BI, McDonald P, et al. The effects of olanzapine on genome-wide DNA methylation in the hippocampus and cerebellum. *Clin Epigenetics*. 2014;6(1):1. doi: 10.1186/1868-7083-6-1.

[6] Consortium C-DG of the PG. Identification of risk loci with shared effects on five major psychiatric disorders: a genome-wide analysis. *Lancet*. 2013;381(9875):1371–1379. doi: 10.1016/S0140-6736(12)62129-1.

[7] Li J, Zhao L, You Y, et al. Schizophrenia related variants in CACNA1C also confer risk of autism. *PLoS One*. 2015;10(7):1–12. doi:10.1371/journal.pone.0133247.

[8] Hui L, Wu JQ, Zhang X, et al. Association between the angiotensin-converting enzyme gene insertion/deletion polymorphism and first-episode patients with schizophrenia in a Chinese Han population. *Hum Psychopharmacol*. 2014;29(3):274–279. doi:10.1002/hup.2396.

[9] Sekar A, Bialas AR, de Rivera H, et al. Schizophrenia risk from complex variation of complement component 4. *Nature*. 2016;530(7589):177–183. doi:10.1038/nature16549.

[10] Jalbrzikowski M, Lazaro MT, Gao F, et al. Transcriptome profiling of peripheral blood in 22q11.2 deletion syndrome reveals functional pathways related to psychosis and autism spectrum disorder. *PLoS One*. 2015;10(7):1–22. doi:10.1371/journal.pone. 0132542.

[11] Jonas RK, Montojo CA, Bearden CE. The 22q11.2 deletion syndrome as a window into complex neuropsychiatric disorders over the lifespan. *Biol Psychiatry*. 2014;75(5):351–360. doi:10.1016/j.biopsych.2013.07.019.

[12] Karayiorgou M, Simon TJ, Gogos JA. 22q11.2 microdeletions: linking DNA structural variation to brain dysfunction and schizophrenia. *Nat Rev Neurosci*. 2010;11(6):402–416. doi:10.1038/nrn2841.

[13] Melka MG, Rajakumar N, O'Reilly R, Singh SM. Olanzapine-induced DNA methylation in the hippocampus and cerebellum in genes mapped to human 22q11 and implicated in schizophrenia. *Psychiatr Genet*. 2014;1–7:25(2):88–94. doi:10.1097/YPG. 0000000000000069.

[14] Egawa J, Hoya S, Watanabe Y, et al. Rare UNC13B variations and risk of schizophrenia: Whole-exome sequencing in a multiplex family and follow-up resequencing and a case-control study. *Am J Med Genet, B: Neuropsychiat Genet*. 2016;171(6):797–805.

[15] Weissensteiner H, Forer L, Fuchsberger C, et al. mtDNA-Server: next-generation sequencing data analysis of human mitochondrial DNA in the cloud. *Nucleic Acids Res*. 2016:gkw247;44:64–69. doi:10.1093/nar/gkw247.

[16] Sequeira A, Rollins B, Magnan C, et al. Mitochondrial mutations in subjects with psychiatric disorders. *PLoS One*. 2015;10(5):1–17. doi:10.1371/journal.pone.0127280.

[17] Razin A, Cedar H. DNA methylation and gene expression. *Microbiol Rev*. 1991;55(3): 451–458. doi:10.1002/wsbm.64.

[18] Bredberg A, Bodmer W. Cytostatic drug treatment causes seeding of gene promoter methylation. *Eur J Cancer*. 2007;43(5):947–954. doi:10.1016/j.ejca.2006.12.003.

[19] Szyf M. Epigenetic therapeutics in autoimmune disease. *Clin Rev Allergy Immunol*. 2010;39(1):62–77. doi:10.1007/s12016-009-8172-8.

[20] Ehninger D, Li W, Fox K, Stryker MP, Silva AJ. Reversing neurodevelopmental disorders in adults. *Neuron*. 2008;60(6):950–960. doi:10.1016/j.neuron.2008.12.007.

[21] Dempster EL, Pidsley R, Schalkwyk LC, et al. Disease-associated epigenetic changes in monozygotic twins discordant for schizophrenia and bipolar disorder. *Hum Mol Genet*. 2011;20(24):4786–4796. doi:10.1093/hmg/ddr416.

[22] Wockner LF, Noble EP, Lawford BR, et al. Genome-wide DNA methylation analysis of human brain tissue from schizophrenia patients. *Transl Psychiatry*. 2014;4(October 2013):e339. doi:10.1038/tp.2013.111.

[23] Mill J, Tang T, Kaminsky Z, et al. Epigenomic profiling reveals DNA-methylation changes associated with major psychosis. *Am J Hum Genet*. 2008;82(3):696–711. doi: 10.1016/j.ajhg.2008.01.008.

[24] Grace AA. Dopamine system dysregulation by the hippocampus: Implications for the pathophysiology and treatment of schizophrenia. *Neuropharmacology*. 2012;62(3):1342–1348. doi:10.1016/j.neuropharm.2011.05.011.

[25] Eisenberg DP, Ianni AM, Wei S-M, et al. Brain-derived neurotrophic factor (BDNF) Val(66)Met polymorphism differentially predicts hippocampal function in medication-free patients with schizophrenia. *Mol Psychiat*. 2013;18(6):713–720. doi:10.1038/mp.2012.187.

[26] Ginovart N, Kapur S. Role of dopamine D2 receptors for antipsychotic activity. *Handb Exp Pharmacol*. 2012;212:27–52. doi:10.1007/978-3-642-25761-2-2.

[27] Jašović-Gašić M, Vuković O, Pantović M, Cvetić T, Marić-Bojović N. Antipsychotics--history of development and field of indication, new wine--old glassess. *Psychiatr Danub*. 2012;24(Suppl 3):S342–S344. http://www.ncbi.nlm.nih.gov/pubmed/23114814.

[28] Dratcu L, Grandison A, McKay G, Bamidele A, Vasudevan V. Clozapine-resistant psychosis, smoking, and caffeine: managing the neglected effects of substances that our patients consume every day. *Am J Ther*. 2007;14(3):314–318. doi:10.1097/01.pap.0000249958.96498.ce.

[29] Razin A, Kantor B. DNA methylation in epigenetic control of gene expression. *Prog Mol Subcell Biol*. 2005;38:151–167. http://www.ncbi.nlm.nih.gov/pubmed/15881894.

[30] Feng W, Dong Z, He B WK. Analysis method of epigenetic DNA methylation to dynamically investigate the functional activity of transcription factors in gene expression. *BMC Genomics*. 2012;3(532):164-13-532.

[31] Starnawska A, Demontis D MA et al. Hypomethylation of FAM63B in bipolar disorder patients. *Clin Epigenetics*. 2016;8(52):1–6.

[32] Kozlenkov A, Roussos P, Timashpolsky A, et al. Differences in DNA methylation between human neuronal and glial cells are concentrated in enhancers and non-CpG sites. *Nucleic Acids Res*. 2014;42(1):109–127. doi:10.1093/nar/gkt838.

[33] Iwamoto K, Bundo M, Ueda J, et al. Neurons show distinctive DNA methylation profile and higher interindividual variations compared with non-neurons. *Genome Res*. 2011;21(5):688–696. doi:10.1101/gr.112755.110.

[34] Van Den Oord, Clark SXL, et al. A whole methylome CpG-SNP association study of psychosis in blood and brain tissue. *Schizophr Bull*. 2016;42(4):1018–1026.

[35] Walton E, Hass J, Liu J, et al. Correspondence of DNA methylation between blood and brain tissue and its application to schizophrenia research. *Schizophr Bull.* 2015;42(2):sbv074. doi:10.1093/schbul/sbv074.

[36] Shimizu H, Iwayama Y, Yamada K, et al. Genetic and expression analyses of the STOP (MAP6) gene in schizophrenia. *Schizophr Res.* 2006;84(2–3):244–252. doi:10.1016/j.schres.2006.03.017.

[37] Mueller D, Fonseka T, Tiwari A, et al. The role of genetic variation across IL-1 beta, IL-2, IL-6 and BDNF in antipsychotic-induced weight gain. *Neuropsychopharmacology.* 2014;39:S431–S432. doi:10.3109/15622975.2014.984631.

[38] Ferguson-Smith AC. Genomic imprinting: the emergence of an epigenetic paradigm. *Nat Rev Genet.* 2011;12(8):565–575. doi:10.1038/nrg3032.

[39] Heard E, Clerc P, Avner P. X-chromosome inactivation in mammals. *Annu Rev Genet.* 1997;31(1):571–610. doi:10.1146/annurev.genet.31.1.571.

[40] Silva SS, Rowntree RK, Mekhoubad S, Lee JT. X-chromosome inactivation and epigenetic fluidity in human embryonic stem cells. *Proc Natl Acad Sci U S A.* 2008;105(12): 4820–4825. doi:10.1073/pnas.0712136105.

[41] Pai AA, Bell JT, Marioni JC, Pritchard JK, Gilad Y. A genome-wide study of DNA methylation patterns and gene expression levels in multiple human and chimpanzee tissues. *PLoS Genet.* 2011;7(2):1–11. doi:10.1371/journal.pgen.1001316.

[42] Laufer BI, Mantha K, Kleiber ML, Diehl EJ, Addison SMF, Singh SM. Long-lasting alterations to DNA methylation and ncRNAs could underlie the effects of fetal alcohol exposure in mice. *Dis Model Mech.* 2013;6(4):977–992. doi:10.1242/dmm.010975.

[43] Muers M. Gene expression: Disentangling DNA methylation. *Nat Rev Genet.* 2013;14(8): 519. doi:10.1038/nrg3535.

[44] Davies MN, Volta M, Pidsley R, et al. Functional annotation of the human brain methylome identifies tissue-specific epigenetic variation across brain and blood. *Genome Biol.* 2012;13(6):R43. doi:10.1186/gb-2012-13-6-r43.

[45] Ohgane J, Yagi S, Shiota K. Epigenetics: The DNA methylation profile of tissue-dependent and differentially methylated regions in cells. *Placenta.* 2008;29(Suppl.):29–35. doi:10.1016/j.placenta.2007.09.011.

[46] Castellani CA, Melka MG, Diehl EJ, Laufer BI, O'Reilly RL, Singh SM. DNA methylation in psychosis: insights into etiology and treatment. *Epigenomics.* 2015;7(1):67–74. doi: 10.2217/epi.14.66.

[47] Melka MG, Castellani CA, Rajakumar N, O'Reilly R, Singh SM. Olanzapine-induced methylation alters cadherin gene families and associated pathways implicated in psychosis. *BMC Neurosci.* 2014;15:112. doi:10.1186/1471-2202-15-112.

[48] Melka MG, Castellani CA, Laufer BI, Rajakumar RN, O'Reilly R, Singh SM. Olanzapine induced DNA methylation changes support the dopamine hypothesis of psychosis. *J Mol psychiatry*. 2013;1(1):19. doi:10.1186/2049-9256-1-19.

[49] Braff DL. The importance of endophenotypes in schizophrenia research. *Schizophr Res*. 2015;163(1–3):1–8. doi:10.1016/j.schres.2015.02.007.

[50] Melka MG, Castellani CA, O'Reilly R, Singh SM. Insights into the origin of DNA methylation differences between monozygotic twins discordant for schizophrenia. *J Mol Psychiatry*. 2015;3(1):7. doi:10.1186/s40303-015-0013-5.

[51] Gutierrez-Arcelus M, Lappalainen T, Montgomery SB, et al. Passive and active DNA methylation and the interplay with genetic variation in gene regulation. *Elife*. 2013;2013(2):1–18. doi:10.7554/eLife.00523.

[52] Wagner JR, Busche S, Ge B, Kwan T, Pastinen T, Blanchette M. The relationship between DNA methylation, genetic and expression inter-individual variation in untransformed human fibroblasts. *Genome Biol*. 2014;15(2):R37. doi:10.1186/gb-2014-15-2-r37.

[53] Bell JT, Pai AA, Pickrell JK, et al. DNA methylation patterns associate with genetic and gene expression variation in HapMap cell lines. *Genome Biol*. 2011;12(1):R10. doi: 10.1186/gb-2011-12-1-r10.

Chapter 3

Transcriptome Analysis of Systems Biology for Schizophrenia

Kuo-Chuan Huang, Theresa Tsun-Hui Tsao,
Tse-Yi Wang and Sheng-An Lee

Additional information is available at the end of the chapter

http://dx.doi.org/10.5772/66864

Abstract

Transcriptome analysis of postmortem brain samples provides more insights to evaluate biological dysfunctions by analysis of differential expression and genetic interactions in schizophrenia. The growing development of new technologies such as next-generation sequencing (NGS) helps to explore detailed and underlying molecular changes from global perspective of view, not only focus in single SNP variants. It is implicated that schizophrenia genetic and protein interactions may give rise to biological dysfunction not only in dopamine dysfunction but also in immune, energy metabolism, mitochondrial dysfunction and hemostasis. Epigenetic investigation of schizophrenia provides important information on how the environmental factors affect the genetic architecture of the disease. DNA methylation plays a pivotal role in etiology for schizophrenia. The schizophrenia differential methylation genes and differential expression genes were analyzed to find the potential protein complexes related to the etiology of schizophrenia from alteration of DNA methylation. The protein complexes and pathways involved in schizophrenia differential methylation network may be responsible for the etiology and potential treatment targets. It is implicated that the interaction between differential expression candidate genes and differential methylation genes may describe the global view of disease mechanisms and it has important roles in the pathogenesis for schizophrenia.

Keywords: systems biology, protein complexes, methylation, pathway enrichment analysis, network analysis, schizophrenia, epigenetics, mitochondria

1. Introduction

Schizophrenia is a debilitating brain disorder. It belongs to a group of multiple pathologies and is also known as a complex genetic disorder effected or stimulated by environmental factors. Evidences of gene variations as risk factors of schizophrenia have been accumulated since 1938 [1]. Many studies have attempted to resolve the biological and genetic complexity of schizophrenia. However, the molecular mechanism of schizophrenia pathophysiology is far from clear, partly because the disease mechanism mainly locates in brain regions and sampling affected tissues are hence difficult.

The development of treatment is progressing slowly. Mostly antipsychotics are based on the dopamine, serotonin, and γ-Aminobutyric acid (GABA) theory. But none of the theories is conclusive for the disease mechanism. The major treatment of schizophrenia, called the antipsychotics, mostly block corresponding receptors in dopaminergic, serotoninergic, and GABAergic pathways. However, both traditional and atypical antipsychotics have predominant and unneglectable side effects such as involuntary movement disorders and metabolic syndrome. Besides, these medications may not get into the core targets of schizophrenia. Novel treatment strategies have long been anticipated to have more advanced and specific approaches and mechanisms.

New technologies such as next-generation sequencing (NGS), mRNA microarray, high-throughput single nucleotide polymorphism (SNP), and copy number variation (CNV) associations with diseases allowed us to propose novel candidate genes or molecular etiology of mental disorders [2]. Furthermore, the most comprehensive biological databases for schizophrenia genetic research including SZGene [3] and SZGene database (SZDB) [4] have been constructed. The SZGene database (last updated 23 December 2011) has listed 1727 studies investigating over 1008 candidate genes, 8788 polymorphisms, and 287 meta-analysis. In these extensive studies, one or more genetic markers in genes are hypothesized to be involved in the etiology of schizophrenia. SZDB (http://www.szdb.org/) is a comprehensive resource for SZ research which includes SZ genetic data, gene expression data, network-based data, brain expression quantitative trait loci (eQTL) data, and SNP function annotation information. It contains 9,444,230 SNPs with sample size of 82,315, including 35,476 schizophrenia cases and 46,839 controls. Recent NGS researches including comprehensive and collective postmortem brain sample data come from [5].

On the basis of current empirical evidence and mostly consensual assessments of informed opinion, it appears that the historical candidate gene literature did not yield clear insights into the genetic basis of schizophrenia [6].

The schizophrenia-associated studies have difficulties to conclude a simple disease etiology. The important candidate genes varied in literature reviews with low reproducibility. Our group has expanded the association interaction of these candidate genes by constructing genetic association network. It could represent the whole interaction paths by its association trace. Till today, pathway analyses did not enrich smaller ISC p values in hypothesis-driven candidate genes, nor did a comprehensive evaluation of meta-hypotheses driving candidate gene selection. The hypothesis-driven candidate genes studied in the literature are not found enriched for the common genetic variation involved in the etiology of schizophrenia [7]. Functional enrichment analysis is used to identify groups of genes or protein complexes which are differentially expressed in a large set of gene classes. They may have association with disease phenotypes. Statistical approaches help to identify significantly enriched groups of candidate gene. NGS and microarray genome-wide association study (GWAS) results could identify hundreds or thousands of candidate genes for analysis. Specific groups of multiple genes may link to a specific biological pathway, and the simultaneous change in expression level within genes may lead to the difference in phenotypic expression.

2. Next-generation sequencing analysis for mental disorders

2.1. Tissue sample

Different tissue samples obtained from cell culture, blood, postmortem brain, and even cerebrospinal fluid (CSF) have been used to understand the pathology of schizophrenia. The identities of the most significantly dysregulated genes were mostly distinct for each tissue; however, the findings also indicated common biological functions and regulatory pathways or complexes. For example, increased levels of cytokines and correlated N-methyl-D-aspartate (NMDA) receptor change could be found in the peripheral blood and cerebrospinal fluid of schizophrenic patients [8, 9]. In addition, the phenotypic insights of iPSC models in schizophrenia include transcriptional dysregulation, oxidative stress synaptic dysregulation, and neurodevelopmental abnormalities [10], which might be associated and compatible with the antioxidative activity of antipsychotics such as olanzapine and clozaril [11].

In recent years, the postmortem brain tissues from schizophrenia subjects have been extensively studied, which serve as a vital component for illustrating the molecular change of schizophrenia. There are some researches using CSF as a target for analysis of specific gene expression such as immune system or cytokines [8].

2.2. STEA and schizophrenia

Schizophrenic transcriptome enrichment analysis (STEA) can be used to understand the network and pathways for schizophrenia from a global and comprehensive approach. Schizophrenia is a multi-genetic and inheritable disorder. Its onset and etiology involves many genes with interaction of multiple pathways, as well as the interaction of methylation genes with environmental factors or epigenetic insult. For instance, epigenetic changes, like DNA methylation and histone modification, are affected by the environment factors such as stress, chemical, and oxidative reaction.

DNA methylation is the most well-studied epigenetic change and was recently analyzed using STEA in relation to schizophrenia-associated phenotype. Researchers ranked top candidate genes for their correlation between methylation patterns and differential expression level in each of the phenotypes. This system biology approach might prove promising to look for an enrichment of genes and important implications for the disease mechanism that are predicted to be targeted in the progression of the disease.

2.3. Next-generation sequencing

As the high-throughput DNA sequencing technologies are becoming more affordable, the application of these technologies is expected to discover new genomic variations associated within a wide variety of mental disorders. They are also regarded as the key to comprehending those of multivariate genetic origins. The use of next-generation sequencing technologies is expected to facilitate the discovery of schizophrenia candidate genes. In comparison with traditional sequencing, the use of NGS is regarded as an ideal to discover genetic mutations and differential gene expression.

Next-generation sequencing (NGS) is a revolutionized sequencing technique; it makes 6–20 million reads from human genome into pieces at unprecedented speeds to discover novel biological applications. The use of NGS has made possible to identify genetic mutations in complex diseases. NGS is contributing to a new understanding of these diseases, albeit from a different perspective, and thus a new type of research consent is needed. There are different NGS platforms including SOLiD, Illumina, GS Junior System, Pacific Biosciences, and more. NGS data in psychiatric genetic researches face challenges of drastic developments in the understanding mechanisms of schizophrenia. It helps to explore the complex disease from global view aspect, not only in specific SNPs or genetic variants but also the genetic interactions and corresponding networks and pathways.

2.4. The new research models for schizophrenia

The thorough understanding of the potential etiology and pathology of schizophrenia is essential to rapidly improve its diagnoses and more effective therapies. By the understanding of epigenetic changes, gene-gene interaction network using systems biology approaches makes it possible to approach the mechanism of schizophrenia. New analytical technologies such as next-generation sequencing, IPSC neuron model, SZDB, expression pattern analysis, and protein-protein interaction analysis are promising approaches to provide novel insights of pathology which may lead to new treatment strategies for schizophrenia [12]. These approaches may lead to the discovery of underlying epigenetic and genetic factors for schizophrenia and may thereby identify corresponding complexes or pathways and reveal novel therapeutic targets for this devastating disorder [13].

The next-generation data of RNA sequences by big data analysis could bring new insights into the comprehensive and global view and revealed more detailed transcriptional alteration in schizophrenia. Recent developments of DNA sequencing technology and whole genome studies implicated that mutations play a vital role in the genetic architecture of schizophrenia and implicated in several molecular pathways, including chromatin regulation, activity-regulated cytoskeleton, postsynaptic density, and N-methyl-D-aspartate (NMDA) receptor, which are associated with schizophrenia [14]. Schizophrenia-network pathway complex analysis (SCZ-NPCA) has included enrichment analysis which demonstrates the role of the implicated pathways in schizophrenia, such as transcription activity, signaling pathway, cancer-related pathway, tumor suppression, coagulation, insulin secretion, cell cycle, cell differentiation, and apoptosis [5].

2.5. Epigenetics and DNA methylation profiles in schizophrenia

External factors such as environmental stress are known to cause the onset of schizophrenia. Exposure to stress induces stable changes by transcriptional dysfunction, resulting in aberrant changes of genetic expression, neural circuit functions, and ultimately behavior changes and disease symptoms [15]. Epigenetic factors such as aberrant DNA methylation have important roles in regulating gene expression [16]. Epigenetic changes may be one of the pivotal features of many human mental disorders.

Methylation of genomic DNA could mediate gene expression. Although there are no specific methylated gene patterns identified in schizophrenia, there are significant associations between promoter CpG islands (CGI) hypermethylation with gene repression and CGI hypomethylation with increased gene expression [17]. CGIs have been suggested to suppress gene expression by blocking the promoters. Recent researches focus on methylation array in postmortem brain studies such as hypermethylation of *RELN,* hypermethylation and downregulated transcription of *SOX10,* and hypomethylation of *MB-COMT* in promoter [18]. Methylation gene discovery in schizophrenia including COMT, REELIN, dopaminergic, serotonergic, and GABAergic pathways shows differential methylation profiles in schizophrenia [19]. Global hypomethylation has also been noted in schizophrenia patients in experiments with larger sample sizes [20].

Previous studies were mostly done on mouse models or stem cell lines [21, 22]. Nonetheless, a vast amount of methylation arrays of postmortem human brains have been released recently [23, 24]. These latest advances may implicate the importance of methylation patterns in schizophrenic patients. Previous researches of genetic methylation of mental disorders focus on the descriptive finding of differential methylation patterns. But how differentially methylated susceptible genes affect the expression levels of target genes remains to be further systematically analyzed. The relationship between the genetic differential methylation levels and differential expression patterns was explored in schizophrenia. They could be identified as disease biomarkers.

Recent researches gradually focus on novel methylation profile of susceptible genes by network biology analysis. There have been many studies focusing on the discovery of differential expression of schizophrenic candidate genes and the construction of PPI networks and related pathways for the hope of a better understanding of schizophrenia [5, 25–28]. Differentially expressed disease genes from postmortem brain samples of schizophrenia reveal the overall relationships between maker genes and schizophrenia. The constructed disease network and underlying pathways, protein complexes, provided the potential treatment strategy for schizophrenia. It could be proposed as potential targets for developing new treatments due to their functional and topological significance [26].

Analyses of DNA methylation identified potential biological processes that regulate gene expression and contribute to disease mechanisms. We constructed the differential methylation and expression networks to interactions of methylated genes. Therefore, large-scale analyses for differential methylation of schizophrenic susceptible genes were conducted and integrated with the differential expression data of schizophrenic susceptible genes to build the methylation-to-expression genetic network. The network explored the epigenetic mechanism of schizophrenic methylation networks, differential methylation pathways, complexes, and corresponding biological functions. The genetic, epigenetic, and transcriptomic information was integrated to give a comprehensive overview of schizophrenia.

The schizophrenic differential methylation network (SDMN) was constructed for the comprehensive view of methylation profile in schizophrenia. The SDMN was generated by query-query protein-protein interaction (QQPPI) [29] and genetic interactions in Pathway

Commons database of schizophrenic differential methylation genes (SDMGs) [30]. Pathway Commons database [30] which collects BIND [31], BioGRID [32], CTD [33], DIP [34], HPRD [35], HumanCyc [36], IntAct [37], KEGG [38], NetPath [39], PANTHER [40], PhosphoSitePlus [41], PID [42], Reactome [43], SMPDB [44], TRANSFAC [45], MiRTarBase [46], DrugBank [47], Recon 2 [48], and WikiPathways databases [49] contain 34,661 molecular pathways.

The regulatory relations for genetic interactions or the potential pathways may be responsible for disease mechanism of schizophrenia. The differentially expressed genes in the BA22 brain samples of schizophrenia are proposed as schizophrenia candidate marker genes (SCZCGs) [5]. For the exploration of modulation and regulation relations between schizophrenic hypermethylated promotors and differential expression genes, we analyzed hypermethylation promotors and extended protein-protein interactions (PPIs) of SCZCGs to their level one interactions to construct the hypermethylation to differential expression networks (HyDEN).

There are 688 (39.6%) genes (16 hypermethylated/672 hypomethylated, ratio 2.38%) differentially methylated in promotor regions from total 1,869 schizophrenic differentially methylated genes. 639 (36.9%) genes (24 hypermethylated/615 hypomethylated, ratio 3.90%) are differentially methylated in intron. 481 (27.7%) genes (23 hypermethylated/458 hypomethylated, ratio 5.02%) are differentially methylated in exon region. The Venn diagram revealed the most differential methylation genes appear in promotor regions (39.6%) and least differentially methylated in exon regions (27.7%) of the schizophrenic methylation profile on specific gene location. It is indicated that the highly differential methylation in promotor regions may be one of the etiologies for schizophrenia. Recent researches focus on evidences of epigenetic profile of common genetic variants in schizophrenia. In the epigenetic profile of DNA methylation, the phenomena of predominant hypomethylation in promotors were noted in schizophrenia.

The ten schizophrenic hypermethylation genes discovered by SDMN are founded to be associated with biological functions such as cell structure, energy metabolism, mitochondrial function, GABA metabolism, signaling transduction, and zinc finger functions. The influence of schizophrenic hypermethylation genes may play a vital role in the etiology of schizophrenia. The previous studies have validated the relationships between the hypermethylation genes and schizophrenia, yet, little is known about how methylation profile modulates the disease phenotype. By the analysis of SDMN, we could investigate the relationship between the hypermethylation genes and epigenetic mechanism in which the future experimental validation was needed. It may be one of the important disease mechanisms which are responsible for pathogenesis of schizophrenia.

2.6. Potential complexes and pathways for schizophrenia

How does the disease affect human body? Or how does schizophrenia affect the performance of brain? Pathway analysis is the building process of identifying protein interactions, associated annotation, and domain knowledgebase [50]. The pathway enrichment analysis was performed with PID [42], Reactome [51], Cell-Map [30], and HumanCyc [52] databases to obtain the potential pathways for the pathophysiology of schizophrenia. Pathways reported to be associated with pathogenesis of schizophrenia include apoptosis [53], immune system [54], TNF signaling pathways [55], hemostasis [56], p53 pathway [57], BARD1 signaling pathway [58], ceramide signaling pathway [59], ErbB2 signaling pathway [60], and androgen receptor pathway [61] and HDAC signaling pathway [62, 63].

Recent research focuses on the methylation gene groups interact with differential expression gene groups to explore the integrated biological pathways designated to reveal disease pathways discovered in systems biology research which may implicate the mechanism of schizophrenia. External factors such as environmental stress are known to cause the onset of schizophrenia. Exposure to stress induces stable changes by transcriptional dysfunction, resulting in aberrant changes of genetic expression, neural circuit functions, and ultimately behavior changes and disease symptoms [15].

Epigenetic factors such as aberrant DNA methylation have important roles in regulating gene expression [16]. Epigenetic changes may be one of the pivotal features of many human mental disorders. The pathway enrichment analysis may indicate the biological functions influenced by SDMGs. It could reveal the potential disease mechanism and novel therapeutic strategy for schizophrenia.

There are corresponding pathways found in enrichment analysis from SDMGs which may implicate the underlying disease mechanisms and characteristics for schizophrenia under the regulatory role of SDMGs. Top-ranked pathways with FDR p-value <0.05 are TGF beta receptor, pyrimidine metabolism, metabolic pathways, Wnt pathway, folate biosynthesis, nicotinate and nicotinamide metabolism, and purine metabolism.

In order to understand the involved protein complexes in schizophrenia of how SDMGs interact with the expression level of SCZCGs, we searched the comprehensive resource of mammalian protein complexes (CORUM) [64] for the potential protein complexes responsible for the regulation and epigenetic mechanism in schizophrenia. The clique and complex analysis was performed with data of the CORUM database which has a collection of experimentally verified mammalian protein complexes to reveal the corresponding clique complexes. The gene groups from SDMGs and SCZCGs were analyzed and searched against CORUM to find the potential protein complexes related to the etiology of schizophrenia from alteration of DNA methylation. The most important protein complexes involved in SDMGs and SCZCGs may include Nop56p-associated pre-rRNA complex, ribosome-related subunit, mitochondrial respiratory chain complex I, TATA-binding protein-free TAF-II-containing complex (TFTC complex), and P300/CBP-associated factor complex (PCAF complex).

The biological functions of those complexes are associated with ribosome biosynthesis, mitochondrial dysfunction, and pre-rRNA processing. However, the top-ranked complexes represented in SDMGs include SRB/MED-containing cofactor complex (SMCC complex), mediator complex, Nop56p-associated pre-rRNA complex, CDC5L complex, CF IIAm complex, and 55S mitochondrial ribosome complex [65]. These complexes are translated by aberrant SDMGs to perform specific protein functions, which might be the potential molecular mechanism in epigenetic regulation for schizophrenia. The inheritable alterations of these complexes might explain the roles of hereditary factors in the etiology of schizophrenia with DNA methylation

[66]. In cancer etiology, the promoter hypermethylation also plays a major role by aberrant transcription of critical regulator genes such as tumor suppressor genes with the implications for the hypomethylation factors in the novel treatment strategy of cancer [67].

Epigenetic mechanism produces DNA methylation which alters gene expression without altering underlying DNA sequence. *Epigenetic changes may be passed on for multiple generations by cell division* [68]. Evidences of linkage analysis in schizophrenic family suggest a hereditary susceptibility [69]. The methylation of DNA confers long-term epigenetic silencing which could be reprogrammed by demethylation of DNA repair [70]. It is implicated that the epigenetic change, especially from the differentially expression genes, regulates the methylation of SDMGs and the production of corresponding protein complexes.

Recent study suggests that the hypomethylated genes are predominant in schizophrenia. Reducing hypomethylation of SDMGs or SCZCGs could be a novel therapeutic treatment method for schizophrenia. There might be the protective factors as per the etiology of cancer [25], in which most promotors are hypermethylated. Some hypermethylating agent, such as vitamin B1, induces upregulation of methyltransferase and reversion of hypomethylation as an adjuvant treatment in schizophrenia [71]. It has postulated that deficiency of vitamin B1 may result in genetic methylation and biochemical lesion relating to neurotransmitter metabolism in the brain, leading to psychotic manifestations [72].

2.7. Mitochondrial dysfunction in schizophrenia by genetic interaction network

By the analysis of transcriptome profiles in postmortem brain tissues and interactions between differential expression candidate genes, the novel finding of potential complexes and pathways could facilitate the investigation of potential schizophrenic pathoetiology. Recent researches focus on theories related to the hypofunction of mitochondria which may contribute to the pathogenesis of schizophrenia, especially negative symptoms such as anhedonia, lack of emotional expression, flattening, poor social and interpersonal activities, and poor self-care. Some advanced techniques propose the replacement of mitochondria; even restoration of mitochondrial function might be potential treatment for alleviation of the negative symptoms of schizophrenia. Since the mitochondria are responsible for vital biological processes such as energy metabolism, calcium buffering, and apoptosis, it indicates the importance of mitochondria dysfunction in the manifestation of schizophrenia [73].

The genetic profile of mitochondria and energy metabolism in the analysis of brain samples may contribute to reveal the novel insight to the etiology of schizophrenia [73, 74]. The genetic interactions and intermediate mediators among mitochondrial genes and many underexpressed SCZCGs indicate the genetic predisposition of mitochondria dysfunction in schizophrenia. The genetic interactions between mitochondria and schizophrenia may be revealed by the DRD2-NDUFS7 and the FLNA-ARRB2 interactions [5].

In SDMG, NDUFA10 has been found to be associated with the abnormalities of mitochondrial function in schizophrenia [75]. It plays a key role in respiratory electron transport chain responded to the exposure of antipsychotics [76]. NDUFA10 mutation causes mitochondrial complex I deficiency. It is associated with the progressive neurodegenerative disease such as

Leigh syndrome [77], which possibly shares the same etiopathogenesis with schizophrenia [78]. The mechanism involving NDUFA10 could be novel targets for schizophrenic therapeutic treatments. BARD1, RBMS1, PRKAB1, UBE2L3, SCO2, PIN4, MRPL43, BAG6, NDUFB11, CAPN1, STAT3, MPST, TCOF1, and SEC24C are all under-expressed genes which interact with the respiratory chain complex I in mitochondria.

3. Novel treatment strategy of antipsychotics

If the SCZCGs are responsible for the gene targets of disease mechanism of schizophrenia, the associated complexes or drugs derived from SCZCGs may contribute to novel treatment for schizophrenia whether they were traditional or atypical antipsychotics related. From the analysis of important cliques in SCZCGs, some of the drugs derived from clique analysis and mapped to the gene targets from DrugBank such as lovastatin and retinoid acid.

Lovastatin, a cholesterol-lowering agent is targeted by HDAC2. It was also the principal statin produced from *Monascus purpureus* derived from red yeast rice [79]. It has been implicated that statins target many of the pathways to neuroprogression in schizophrenia [80]. Adapalene, Tazarotene, and Tamibarotene are retinoids which involved RARA gene with multiple functions including eye vision, immune function, and activation of tumor suppressor genes. Retinoic acid has been reported for the treatment of schizophrenia. More and more evidence regarding retinoid dysregulation in schizophrenia implicated targeting retinoid receptors may be a novel approach to treat schizophrenia [25, 81].

Although there is not yet a clear and well-evidenced disease mechanism for schizophrenia, the current findings may contribute to novel indications or drug repurposing for schizophrenia. However, further evaluation and validation are needed in the near future.

Author details

Kuo-Chuan Huang[1, 2], Theresa Tsun-Hui Tsao[3], Tse-Yi Wang[4] and Sheng-An Lee[5*]

*Address all correspondence to: shengan@mail.knu.edu.tw

1 Department of Psychiatry, Beitou Branch, Tri-Service General Hospital, National Defense Medical Center, Taipei, Taiwan

2 Department of Nursing, Ching Kuo Institute of Management and Health, Keelung, Taiwan

3 Department of Psychiatry, College of Medicine, National Taiwan University Hospital ,Taipei, Taiwan

4 Molecular Anthropology and Transfusion Medicine Research Laboratory, Mackay Memorial Hospital ,Taipei City, Taiwan

5 Department of Information Management, Kainan University, Taoyuan, Taiwan

References

[1] Kallmann, F.J., *The genetics of schizophrenia*. 1938, Oxford, England: J. J. Augustin. xvi, 291.

[2] Gejman, P.V., A.R. Sanders, and J. Duan, *The role of genetics in the etiology of schizophrenia*. Psychiatr Clin North Am, 2010. **33**(1): pp. 35–66.

[3] Allen, N.C., et al., *Systematic meta-analyses and field synopsis of genetic association studies in schizophrenia: the SzGene database*. Nat Genet, 2008. **40**(7): pp. 827–34.

[4] Wu, Y., Y.G. Yao, and X.J. Luo, SZDB: a database for schizophrenia genetic research. Schizophr Bull, 2016 Jul 22. pii: sbw102.

[5] Huang, K.C., et al., *Transcriptome alterations of mitochondrial and coagulation function in schizophrenia by cortical sequencing analysis*. BMC Genom, 2014. **15**(Suppl. 9): p. S6.

[6] Farrell, M.S., et al., *Evaluating historical candidate genes for schizophrenia*. Mol Psychiatry, 2015. **20**(5): pp. 555–62.

[7] Collins, A.L., et al., *Hypothesis-driven candidate genes for schizophrenia compared to genome-wide association results*. Psychol Med, 2012. **42**(3): pp. 607–16.

[8] Schwieler, L., et al., *Increased levels of IL-6 in the cerebrospinal fluid of patients with chronic schizophrenia–significance for activation of the kynurenine pathway*. J Psychiatry Neurosci, 2015. **40**(2): pp. 126–33.

[9] Miller, B.J., et al., *Meta-analysis of cytokine alterations in schizophrenia: clinical status and antipsychotic effects*. Biol Psychiatry, 2011. **70**(7): pp. 663–71.

[10] Jacobs, B.M., *A dangerous method? The use of induced pluripotent stem cells as a model for schizophrenia*. Schizophr Res, 2015. **168**(1-2): pp. 563–8.

[11] Sadowska-Bartosz, I., et al., *Antioxidant properties of atypical antipsychotic drugs used in the treatment of schizophrenia*. Schizophr Res, 2016. **176**(2-3): pp. 245–51.

[12] Rudan, I., *New technologies provide insights into genetic basis of psychiatric disorders and explain their co-morbidity*. Psychiatr Danub, 2010. **22**(2): pp. 190–2.

[13] Schreiber, M., M. Dorschner, and D. Tsuang, *Next-generation sequencing in schizophrenia and other neuropsychiatric disorders*. Am J Med Genet B Neuropsychiatr Genet, 2013. **162B**(7): pp. 671–8.

[14] Kato, T., *Whole genome/exome sequencing in mood and psychotic disorders*. Psychiatry Clin Neurosci, 2015. **69**(2): pp. 65–76.

[15] Nestler, E.J., et al., Epigenetic basis of mental illness. Neuroscientist, 2016 Oct;22(5):447-63.

[16] Lim, D.H.K. and E.R. Maher, *DNA methylation: a form of epigenetic control of gene expression*. Obstet Gynaecol, 2010. **12**(1): pp. 37–42.

[17] Li, Y., et al., *Genome-wide methylome analyses reveal novel epigenetic regulation patterns in schizophrenia and bipolar disorder*. Biomed Res Int, 2015. **2015**: p. 201587.

[18] Nishioka, M., et al., *DNA methylation in schizophrenia: progress and challenges of epigenetic studies*. Genome Med, 2012. **4**(12): p. 96.

[19] Rivollier, F., et al., *Epigenetics of schizophrenia: a review*. Encéphale, 2014. **40**(5): pp. 380–6.

[20] Shimabukuro, M., et al., *Global hypomethylation of peripheral leukocyte DNA in male patients with schizophrenia: a potential link between epigenetics and schizophrenia*. J Psychiatr Res, 2007. **41**(12): pp. 1042–6.

[21] Dong, E., et al., *Behavioral and molecular neuroepigenetic alterations in prenatally stressed mice: relevance for the study of chromatin remodeling properties of antipsychotic drugs*. Transl Psychiatry, 2016. **6**: p. e711.

[22] O'Shea, K.S. and M.G. McInnis, *Neurodevelopmental origins of bipolar disorder: iPSC models*. Mol Cell Neurosci, 2016. **73**: pp. 63–83.

[23] Jaffe, A.E., et al., *Mapping DNA methylation across development, genotype and schizophrenia in the human frontal cortex*. Nat Neurosci, 2016. **19**(1): pp. 40–7.

[24] Hannon, E., et al., *Methylation QTLs in the developing brain and their enrichment in schizophrenia risk loci*. Nat Neurosci, 2016. **19**(1): pp. 48–54.

[25] Huang, K.C., et al., *Analysis of schizophrenia and hepatocellular carcinoma genetic network with corresponding modularity and pathways: novel insights to the immune system*. BMC Genom, 2013. **14** Suppl. 5: p. S10.

[26] Lee, S.A., et al., *Construction and analysis of the protein-protein interaction networks for schizophrenia, bipolar disorder, and major depression*. BMC Bioinform, 2011. **12**(Suppl. 13): p. S20.

[27] Wu, J.Q., et al., *Transcriptome sequencing revealed significant alteration of cortical promoter usage and splicing in schizophrenia*. PLoS One, 2012. **7**(4): p. e36351.

[28] Sun, J., et al., *Schizophrenia gene networks and pathways and their applications for novel candidate gene selection*. PLoS One, 2010. **5**(6): p. e11351.

[29] Lee, S.A., et al., *POINeT: protein interactome with sub-network analysis and hub prioritization*. BMC Bioinform, 2009. **10**: p. 114.

[30] Cerami, E.G., et al., *Pathway Commons, a web resource for biological pathway data*. Nucleic Acids Res, 2011. **39**(Database issue): pp. D685–90.

[31] Bader, G.D., et al., *BIND: the Biomolecular Interaction Network Database*. Nucleic Acids Res, 2001. **29**(1): pp. 242–5.

[32] Stark, C., et al., *BioGRID: a general repository for interaction datasets*. Nucleic Acids Res, 2006. **34**(Database issue): pp. D535–9.

[33] Mattingly, C.J., et al., *The Comparative Toxicogenomics Database (CTD): a resource for comparative toxicological studies*. J Exp Zool A Comp Exp Biol, 2006. **305**(9): pp. 689–92.

[34] Orchard, S., et al., *Protein interaction data curation: the International Molecular Exchange (IMEx) consortium*. Nat Methods, 2012. **9**(4): pp. 345–50.

[35] Mathivanan, S., et al., *An evaluation of human protein-protein interaction data in the public domain*. BMC Bioinform, 2006. **7**(Suppl. 5): p. S19.

[36] Caspi, R., et al., *The MetaCyc database of metabolic pathways and enzymes and the BioCyc collection of pathway/genome databases*. Nucleic Acids Res, 2012. **40**(Database issue): pp. D742–53.

[37] Orchard, S., et al., *The MIntAct project–IntAct as a common curation platform for 11 molecular interaction databases*. Nucleic Acids Res, 2014. **42**(Database issue): pp. D358–63.

[38] Kanehisa, M., et al., *Data, information, knowledge and principle: back to metabolism in KEGG*. Nucleic Acids Res, 2014. **42**(Database issue): pp. D199–205.

[39] Kandasamy, K., et al., *NetPath: a public resource of curated signal transduction pathways*. Genome Biol, 2010. **11**(1): p. R3.

[40] Thomas, P.D., et al., *PANTHER: a browsable database of gene products organized by biological function, using curated protein family and subfamily classification*. Nucleic Acids Res, 2003. **31**(1): pp. 334–41.

[41] Hornbeck, P.V., et al., *PhosphoSitePlus, 2014: mutations, PTMs and recalibrations*. Nucleic Acids Res, 2015. **43**(Database issue): pp. D512–20.

[42] Schaefer, C.F., et al., *PID: the Pathway Interaction Database*. Nucleic Acids Res, 2009. **37**(Database issue): pp. D674–9.

[43] Croft, D., et al., *Reactome: a database of reactions, pathways and biological processes*. Nucleic Acids Res, 2011. **39**(Database issue): pp. D691–7.

[44] Jewison, T., et al., *SMPDB 2.0: big improvements to the Small Molecule Pathway Database*. Nucleic Acids Res, 2014. **42**(Database issue): pp. D478–84.

[45] Wingender, E., *The TRANSFAC project as an example of framework technology that supports the analysis of genomic regulation*. Brief Bioinform, 2008. **9**(4): pp. 326–32.

[46] Hsu, S.D., et al., *miRTarBase: a database curates experimentally validated microRNA-target interactions*. Nucleic Acids Res, 2011. **39**(Database issue): pp. D163–9.

[47] Law, V., et al., *DrugBank 4.0: shedding new light on drug metabolism*. Nucleic Acids Res, 2014. **42**(Database issue): pp. D1091–7.

[48] Thiele, I., et al., *A community-driven global reconstruction of human metabolism*. Nat Biotechnol, 2013. **31**(5): pp. 419–25.

[49] Kutmon, M., et al., *WikiPathways: capturing the full diversity of pathway knowledge*. Nucleic Acids Res, 2016. **44**(D1): pp. D488–94.

[50] Viswanathan, G.A., et al., *Getting started in biological pathway construction and analysis*. PLoS Comput Biol, 2008. **4**(2): p. e16.

[51] Jupe, S., et al., *Reactome – a curated knowledgebase of biological pathways: megakaryocytes and platelets*. J Thromb Haemost, 2012. **10**(11): pp. 2399–402.

[52] Romero, P., et al., *Computational prediction of human metabolic pathways from the complete human genome*. Genome Biol, 2005. **6**(1): p. R2.

[53] Boiadzhian, A.S., et al., *Markers of apoptotic dysfunction in schizophrenia*. Mol Biol (Mosk), 2013. **47**(4): pp. 674–80.

[54] de Witte, L., et al., Cytokine alterations in first-episode schizophrenia patients before and after antipsychotic treatment. Schizophr Res, 2014 Apr;154(1–3):23–9.

[55] Paredes, R.M., et al., *Metabolomic profiling of schizophrenia patients at risk for metabolic syndrome*. Int J Neuropsychopharmacol, 2014: pp. 1–10.

[56] Dietrich-Muszalska, A. and B. Olas, *The changes of aggregability of blood platelets in schizophrenia*. World J Biol Psychiatry, 2009. **10**(2): pp. 171–6.

[57] Lajin, B., et al., *Association between polymorphisms in the genes for tumor suppressor protein p53 and its regulator NAD(P)H: quinone oxidoreductase 1 (NQO1) and schizophrenia in a Syrian study cohort*. Arch Med Res, 2013. **44**(2): pp. 121–6.

[58] van Schijndel, J.E., et al., *Three-cohort targeted gene screening reveals a non-synonymous TRKA polymorphism associated with schizophrenia*. J Psychiatr Res, 2009. **43**(15): pp. 1195–9.

[59] Smesny, S., et al., *Skin ceramide alterations in first-episode schizophrenia indicate abnormal sphingolipid metabolism*. Schizophr Bull, 2013. **39**(4): pp. 933–41.

[60] Kanakry, C.G., et al., *Neuregulin-1 regulates cell adhesion via an ErbB2/phosphoinositide-3 kinase/Akt-dependent pathway: potential implications for schizophrenia and cancer*. PLoS One, 2007. **2**(12): p. e1369.

[61] Tsai, S.J., et al., *Distribution of androgen receptor CAG repeat polymorphism in Chinese schizophrenia and its correlation with age at onset*. Psychoneuroendocrinology, 2006. **31**(2): pp. 270–4.

[62] Han, H., et al., *Associations of histone deacetylase-2 and histone deacetylase-3 genes with schizophrenia in a Chinese population*. Asia Pac Psychiatry, 2013. **5**(1): pp. 11–6.

[63] Kim, T., et al., *Association of histone deacetylase genes with schizophrenia in Korean population*. Psychiatry Res, 2010. **178**(2): pp. 266–9.

[64] Ruepp, A., et al., *CORUM: the comprehensive resource of mammalian protein complexes*. Nucleic Acids Res, 2008. **36**(Database issue): pp. D646–50.

[65] Lee, S.A. and K.C. Huang, *Epigenetic profiling of human brain differential DNA methylation networks in schizophrenia*. BMC Medical Genomics, 2016. **9**(Suppl. X): p. S2, (In press).

[66] Roth, T.L., et al., *Epigenetic mechanisms in schizophrenia*. Biochim Biophys Acta, 2009. **1790**(9): pp. 869–77.

[67] Baylin, S.B., *DNA methylation and gene silencing in cancer*. Nat Clin Pract Oncol, 2005. **2**(Suppl. 1): pp. S4–11.

[68] Bird, A., *Perceptions of epigenetics*. Nature, 2007. **447**(7143): pp. 396–8.

[69] Paunio, T., et al., *Linkage analysis of schizophrenia controlling for population substructure*. Am J Med Genet B Neuropsychiatr Genet, 2009. **150B**(6): pp. 827–35.

[70] Reik, W., *Stability and flexibility of epigenetic gene regulation in mammalian development*. Nature, 2007. **447**(7143): pp. 425–32.

[71] Ghufran, M.S., K. Ghosh, and S.R. Kanade, *Aflatoxin B1 induced upregulation of protein arginine methyltransferase 5 in human cell lines*. Toxicon, 2016. **119**: pp. 117–21.

[72] Osiezagha, K., et al., *Thiamine deficiency and delirium*. Innov Clin Neurosci, 2013. **10**(4): pp. 26–32.

[73] Karry, R., E. Klein, and D. Ben Shachar, *Mitochondrial complex I subunits expression is altered in schizophrenia: a postmortem study*. Biol Psychiatry, 2004. **55**(7): pp. 676–84.

[74] Martins-de-Souza, D., et al., *Proteome analysis of schizophrenia patients Wernicke's area reveals an energy metabolism dysregulation*. BMC Psychiatry, 2009. **9**: p. 17.

[75] Park, C. and S.K. Park, *Molecular links between mitochondrial dysfunctions and schizophrenia*. Mol Cells, 2012. **33**(2): pp. 105–10.

[76] Ji, B., et al., *A comparative proteomics analysis of rat mitochondria from the cerebral cortex and hippocampus in response to antipsychotic medications*. J Proteome Res, 2009. **8**(7): pp. 3633–41.

[77] Hoefs, S.J., et al., *NDUFA10 mutations cause complex I deficiency in a patient with Leigh disease*. Eur J Hum Genet, 2011. **19**(3): pp. 270–4.

[78] Mnif, L., R. Sellami, and J. Masmoudi, *Schizophrenia and Leigh syndrome, a simple comorbidity or the same etiopathogeny: about a case*. Pan Afr Med J, 2015. **22**: p. 333.

[79] Dikshit, R. and P. Tallapragada, *Bio-synthesis and screening of nutrients for lovastatin by Monascus sp. under solid-state fermentation*. J Food Sci Technol, 2015. **52**(10): pp. 6679–86.

[80] Ghanizadeh, A., et al., *Lovastatin for the adjunctive treatment of schizophrenia: a preliminary randomized double-blind placebo-controlled trial*. Psychiatry Res, 2014. **219**(3): pp. 431–5.

[81] Lerner, V., P.J. McCaffery, and M.S. Ritsner, *Targeting retinoid receptors to treat schizophrenia: rationale and progress to date*. CNS Drugs, 2016. **30**(4): pp. 269–80.

Chapter 4

Toxoplasma gondii and Schizophrenia: A Relationship That Is Not Ruled Out

Antonio Sorlozano-Puerto and
Jose Gutierrez-Fernandez

Additional information is available at the end of the chapter

http://dx.doi.org/10.5772/66018

Abstract

Over recent years, it has been proposed that some diseases of unknown origin, such as schizophrenia, may be caused by persistent chronic infections coupled with a genetic component and may be perpetuated by the immune system. This hypothesis is supported by epidemiological and biological evidence on the exposure of schizophrenics to infectious diseases during prenatal or postnatal periods, including *Toxoplasma gondii*, chlamydia, human herpes virus, human endogenous retroviruses, parvovirus B19, mumps, and flu viruses. This growing list of microbes will undoubtedly continue to increase in the future. Linking infection to schizophrenia is a complex challenge that requires further experimental and epidemiological research. *T. gondii* is the infectious agent that has most frequently been related to neuropsychiatric disorders, including schizophrenia, and it is considered to represent a highly useful model to analyze the influence of a microorganism on human behavior and the development of psychiatric disease. It may also help to detect patient subpopulations susceptible to treatment with specific antimicrobials by improving definition of the differential phenotype of the disease, and it offers the possibility of a preventive approach.

Keywords: schizophrenia, *Toxoplasma gondii*, antibodies, behavior, cytokine, neurotransmitter, gene-infection interaction

1. Introduction

Over the past few years, it has been proposed by some authors that schizophrenia may be caused by central nervous system (CNS) disorders during neurodevelopment (i.e., congenital) or during the postnatal period, at least in some patient subgroups [1]. These disorders may be related to environmental exposure to toxic products, radiation, stress, fetal hypoxia, nutritional problems, infections (especially when chronic and persistent), and/or, according to more recent data, gut microbiota [2, 3]. Any of these exposures could possibly affect cognitive functions and behavior patterns with important neuropsychiatric consequences, including irreversible neurological lesions leading to neuronal dysfunction, behavior problems, mental retardation, learning difficulties, or mood disorders [4–9]. Participation by microbial agents in the development of schizophrenia is suggested by medical evidence, with prenatal or perinatal infection being the most frequent cause of severe congenital malformations and mental impairment [10]. Their involvement is also supported by epidemiological evidence on the exposure of schizophrenic patients to *T. gondii*, chlamydia, human herpes virus, human endogenous retroviruses, parvovirus B19, and rubella, mumps, or influenza viruses, among other microorganisms [11].

According to current pathogenic models, microorganisms may produce various inflammatory and/or immunological disorders in the infected brain, giving rise to neurotransmitter synthesis disorders with important clinical repercussions [7]. Schizophrenia has been related to the production of inflammatory cytokines that alter the synthesis of dopamine and other neurotransmitters [12] and to fetal neuronal tissue damage due to the transplacental transfer of maternal antibodies, which might underlie development of the disease decades later [13]. This association with inflammatory and immunologic disorders has been observed in studies of animal models and human cells. Thus, maternal infection of mice and rats during pregnancy was associated with behavioral disorders in the offspring that were very similar to those reported in schizophrenic patients. Various studies in murine models revealed an association between prenatal infection and marked deficits in sensory information processing, in the expression of certain neurotransmitters (e.g., dopamine) and of cytokines, and in the immune function, all of which emerged in the offspring. Their onset is at an age equivalent to human adolescence and is earlier, with more severe effects, in male *versus* female rats, and these alterations can be reverted by the administration of antipsychotic drugs. In short, the fetus can be damaged by numerous infectious agents, whether or not they are primarily neurotropic, which may favor in a direct or immune-mediated manner the development of neurological damage, disorders in neurotransmitter expression, and modifications in sensory information processing [14].

There is intense and increasing research interest in the relationship between schizophrenia and infectious agents. Irreversible mild or severe neurophysiologic alterations may result from fetal infection, maternal infection with secondary fetal involvement *via* inflammatory and/or immunological mechanisms, or postnatal infection and may lead to the emergence of schizophrenia over the years. The full elucidation of these associations may allow specific antimicrobial treatments to be added to current symptomatic (or antipsychotic) treatments for these patients [5], potentially offering a preventive and curative approach to the disease, given that they would act on known and treatable etiologic factors.

T. gondii is the infectious agent that has most frequently been related to neuropsychiatric disorders, including schizophrenia, and it is considered to represent a useful model to analyze the influence of a microorganism on human behavior and the development of psychiatric disease [15]. It is an obligate intracellular protozoa belonging to the *Coccidia* subclass of the phylum *Apicomplexa* and causes toxoplasmosis. Its definitive hosts are cats and other felines, which

http://dx.doi.org/10.5772/66018

are the only animals in which the sexual stage of their life cycle takes place (in intestines), forming oocysts that are eliminated through the feces. Hot-blooded vertebrates such as birds and other mammals, including humans, are intermediate hosts. Humans can become infected by various pathways, such as: the intake of undercooked meat containing latent forms of the parasite (bradyzoites in tissue cysts), fresh food (e.g., fruit and vegetables), or water contaminated with oocysts from cat feces; blood transfusions; transplantation of solid organ or stem cells, or transplacental transmission. Upon reaching tissues, *T. gondii* rapidly replicates in the form of tachyzoites until tissue proliferation and expansion of the parasite are impeded by the immune response, after which its replication slows and it remains in tissue cysts in latent or bradyzoite form. Cysts are most frequently found in skeletal muscle, myocardium, CNS, and eyes and are responsible for persistent infection [16, 17].

Primary infection usually takes place during childhood, when only a small percentage of people show symptoms, which are mild and include general discomfort, lethargy, cervical lymphadenopathy, and/or eye disease, among others. Most parasitized individuals remain asymptomatic for a long time period, even throughout their life, and host the latent form of *T. gondii*. However, chronic infection can be reactivated in immunocompromised individuals (AIDS, transplanted, and oncology patients, etc.), giving rise to various symptoms and even, in death. This reactivation is often associated with nervous system symptoms, such as Guillain-Barré syndrome, diffuse encephalopathy, meningoencephalitis, or brain abscesses [17, 18]. Human parasitizations, although generally considered asymptomatic, may cause behavioral disorders and the development of a psychiatric disease such as schizophrenia due to damage resulting from the initial infection, from the host immune response to the parasite, or from the persistence of cysts in the CNS [19]. Accordingly, the concept of asymptomatic chronic parasitization is currently under debate [20].

T. gondii is a plausible candidate as an infectious origin of schizophrenia and has attracted considerable research attention for the following reasons: the possibility of its transplacental transmission; its marked neurotropism; its capacity for persistent infection, remaining in latent form but with the possibility of reactivation; its association with brain development disorders and anomalies; its relationship with behavior disorders in animal and human models; and *in vitro* evidence of the inhibition of its growth in cell culture by antipsychotic drugs.

2. Epidemiologic data on the association between toxoplasmosis and schizophrenia

One of the first approaches adopted to explore a possible relationship between *T. gondii* infection and schizophrenia was to analyze epidemiological data on the two diseases. Initial conclusions were as follows:

- Both have a familial incidence. This is explained in the case of schizophrenia by the possible participation of certain genes in its pathogeny [21], and in the case of toxoplasmosis by the possible common exposure of family members to the parasite, although a genetic influence has also been proposed [22].

- There is a relatively high frequency of stillborns among both schizophrenic [23] and parasitized [24] mothers.
- Both diseases typically show a decreased prevalence in geographic areas with small populations of felines [25, 26].
- Initial symptoms in both diseases commonly manifest between the second and third decade of life [27, 28].
- The prevalence of both diseases is higher among populations with lower socioeconomic level and living in overcrowded conditions [29, 30].

These and other published findings indicate that the two diseases have some similar features and may even be epidemiologically related. However, they are inadequate to establish etiological relationships, and a pathophysiological approach is required to explore causality.

3. Studies based on the detection of anti-*Toxoplasma gondii* antibodies

For more than six decades, the relationship between schizophrenia and toxoplasmosis has been explored by studying a specific immune response [31]. Various meta-analyses have demonstrated a significantly higher prevalence of anti-*T. gondii* antibodies in schizophrenic patients than in controls, with odds ratios ranging between 2.7 [11, 32–34] and 1.8 [35].

In the natural time course of toxoplasmosis, IgM antibodies against *T. gondii* are the first to be detected in serum, a few days after infection. These are usually negativized between weeks 4 and 12 but can remain detectable for months or even years in a large number of patients. IgG antibodies are detected at around 2 weeks later than IgM antibodies, reaching a maximum level in the 2nd to 3rd month and persisting throughout life in residual titers. The presence of IgM antibodies in the absence of IgG indicates recent infection, while the presence of IgG indicates chronic infection, especially in the absence of IgM. The reactivation of a persistent infection can be accompanied by increased IgG and/or IgM values, although these antibodies can be undetectable in immunocompromised patients [36].

Most studies have centered on the humoral immune response, comparing anti-*T. gondii* IgG and IgM antibodies between schizophrenic patients (in different clinical/therapeutic situations) and controls. This method is widely employed because of the ease with which samples (usually serum, occasionally cerebrospinal fluid) can be gathered and the high degree of reproducibility, specificity, and sensitivity obtained. Many of these studies reported higher levels of antibodies (IgG and, in some studies, IgM) against *T. gondii* in patients with schizophrenia than in other populations, including patients with a different psychiatric disorder [32, 37–51]. However, findings have been inconsistent [52, 53], and account should be taken of the publication bias against studies without significant results [11].

Clinical manifestations differ between seropositive and seronegative schizophrenic patients, with a predominance in the former of positive symptoms (delirium, hallucinations, disorganized thinking), cognitive disorders (abstract thinking difficulties, disorientation, attention deficit), and agitation [50, 54]. Some researchers also observed that patients with schizophrenia and anti-*T. gondii* antibodies had a significantly higher risk of dying from natural causes [55] and were more likely to attempt suicide [56] in comparison with seronegative patients.

The above studies suggest a strong association between these diseases, with a significantly higher frequency of chronic parasitization in schizophrenic patients than in other population groups. However, if schizophrenia is a consequence of chronic CNS infection, which usually takes place at an early age, the question arises as to why it typically appears between the second and third decades of life. According to Yolken et al. [51], a significant increase in IgG titers observed in patients with a first schizophrenia episode may be compatible with a reactivation of the infection (previously in latent phase) that becomes clinically manifest in the onset of the disease *via* an immune-mediated mechanism. Some authors proposed that the immunoglobulins may cross the blood-brain barrier in this situation and react with brain tissue antigens due to their molecular mimicry with *T. gondii* antigens. This is similar to observations in such autoimmune diseases as systemic lupus erythematosus or in paraneoplastic syndromes [57]. Associations with the presence of anti-*Toxoplasma* IgM are less well documented [35], although Monroe et al. [58] reported in their meta-analysis a significant 1.7-fold greater likelihood of *T. gondii* IgM antibodies in patients with acute psychosis than in controls. It was concluded that *T. gondii* IgM antibodies may indicate either an acute/recent infection or a reinfection, possibly with a different genotype.

However, although a strong association has been described between schizophrenia and parasitization, these studies do not provide evidence to confirm the hypothesis on the infectious etiology of schizophrenia, and a causal relationship has not been demonstrated. Contact with *T. gondii* may be favored by the anomalous behavior, disorganized lifestyle, and/or weaker socioeconomic situation of schizophrenics, with infection being the consequence rather than the cause of their disease, which may explain the positive serological results [50].

4. Seroprevalence studies in mothers and newborns

The possible transplacental transmission of *T. gondii* has attracted considerable attention in seroprevalence studies. Maternal infection during the first or second trimester of pregnancy can lead to severe problems in the offspring, including intracranial calcifications, chorioretinitis, blindness, deafness, hydrocephaly, microcephaly, mental retardation, psychomotor retardation, pancytopenia, or epilepsy. The timing of the transmission is an influential factor: early maternal infection less frequently affects the fetus but is associated with a more severe congenital toxoplasmosis that may result in intrauterine death and miscarriages, while later maternal infection (third trimester) increases the risk of affecting the fetus but is associated with offspring who are asymptomatic [17]. Complications, possibly including schizophrenia, can appear decades later in patients with initially undetected infection due to its reactivation [59].

This type of study can be classified into two groups: those on the presence of antibodies in pregnant women and the development of schizophrenia in their offspring; those on the presence of antibodies in newborns and their later development of schizophrenia. Among the former, Brown et al. [60] and Blomström et al. [61] demonstrated associations between increased anti-*Toxoplasma* IgG levels in pregnant mothers and risk of schizophrenia in their offspring, although other researchers published discrepant results [62]. Xiao et al. [63] observed a significant association between the presence of maternal antibodies against type I *T. gondii* (but not against types II or III) and the onset of psychotic disorders in the offspring. Among the latter group of studies, Mortensen et al. [59] demonstrated that newborn levels of anti-*T. gondii* IgG levels (from the mother) were significantly higher in individuals who developed schizophrenia in adulthood.

Published data suggest that schizophrenia risk in offspring is associated with persistent maternal infection by *T. gondii* but is not directly related to acute maternal infection [64]. If this were the case, a significant association could be expected between the presence of IgM in the serum of mothers and/or newborns and the presence of the disease, which has not been demonstrated [60]. However, this relationship may be masked by the low frequency of anti-*Toxoplasma* IgM detection in pregnant women [24, 65].

As noted above, increased maternal IgG levels can cross the placenta (unlike IgM antibodies) and may damage fetal brain development by molecular mimicry [60, 64]. However, the presence of maternal IgG may indicate a reactivation of latent infection due to the impact of immune system disorders on protozoan replication control during pregnancy [66]; hence, brain development could also be impaired by transplacental transmission and/or the passage of inflammatory cytokines to the fetus [67, 68].

The majority of schizophrenic patients do not have anti-*Toxoplasma* antibodies, and the majority of seropositive patients are not schizophrenic. Therefore, *T. gondii* would only explain a minority of cases. Other factors under investigation that may explain why only some parasitized individuals develop schizophrenia include genetic susceptibility, the infective genotype of the parasite, the existence of different infection pathways, and the timing of toxoplasmosis onset [20, 33, 63].

5. Studies based on *Toxoplasma gondii* nucleic acid detection

Studies of animal brain biopsies have shown *T. gondii* to have high neurotropism, with the capacity to infect glial cells (especially microglia and astrocytes) and neurons, forming persistent cysts in brain tissue [69]. Although no tropism for specific brain regions has been observed, with cysts being detected in many areas, the most frequently parasitized regions are the hippocampus, thalamus, cerebral cortex, cerebellum, olfactory bulb, and, especially, the amygdala [70–73].

However, the presence of brain cysts can only be detected in *postmortem* biopsies, explaining the few studies of this type and the predominance of serological techniques for the detection of chronic infection by *T. gondii* in humans. The presence of glial anomalies, including a reduced amount of astrocytes, has been reported in the brains of schizophrenic patients [74], and it has been speculated that these may possibly result from infection by *T. gondii* [31].

Imaging techniques have revealed a lower density of gray matter in certain brain regions of schizophrenic patients [75], which may be directly related to the infection, given that non-parasitized schizophrenic patients were found to have the same brain morphology as healthy controls [76].

One of the few studies of *postmortem* brain biopsies found no parasite DNA in any subject (14 schizophrenic patients and 26 healthy controls) [77]. There appear to be three possible explanations: first, there was truly no association with the infection; second, the biopsies missed infected brain areas; and finally, the sensitivity of the nucleic acid detection technique might be inadequate. In addition, the detection of parasite DNA only demonstrates the presence of the parasite not its possible effect on the parasitized individual and would not establish an etiological relationship with schizophrenia. Thus, the detection of parasite DNA in brain tissues does not distinguish between asymptomatic patients with latent parasitization and those with encephalitis [17].

A study of blood samples detected parasite DNA in 33 out of 101 samples from schizophrenic patients *versus* 2 out of 55 samples from controls, a significant difference [46]. In contrast, Gutiérrez-Fernández et al. [32] detected parasite DNA in only 1 out of 128 blood samples from schizophrenic patients and in none of 143 samples from controls (nonsignificant difference). However, although the presence of parasite DNA in blood indicates acute infection [17], it does not necessarily signify infection of the brain, and no relationship was found between anti-*Toxoplasma* IgM and schizophrenia in the aforementioned study [46].

6. Studies on behavioral disorders in animals and humans

Research on this issue has included experimental animal studies, mainly in rats and mice. Parasitized animals have shown various behavioral changes, becoming more active, expressing less fear when examining new stimuli, reducing their natural aversion to cat odor or even becoming attracted to it, and demonstrating reduced learning ability and attention or memory deficits [78–83]. According to the "behavioral manipulation hypothesis," these disorders in their intermediate hosts (rodents) represent an evolutionary adaptation of the parasite, facilitating their capture by their definitive host (felines) and completing their life cycle [84, 85]. Although the mechanism by which *T. gondii* induces these behavioral changes is poorly understood, various possibilities have been proposed. It may be due to a direct effect on tissue cysts in specific brain areas such as the amygdala or hippocampus, given that the host response to predator odors was changed by the parasite in male rats infected with *T. gondii* by inducing hypomethylation of the neuropeptide arginine vasopressin in the posterodorsal part of the medial amygdala, an important node of the extrahypothalamic vasopressin system that contains a large number of arginine vasopressin neurons. This epigenetic manipulation produced a greater activation of vasopressinergic neurons after exposure to cat odor, leading to the reversion of fear into attraction [86]. It may also result from the effect of a more diffuse and wider involvement of brain tissues, with no apparent changes, that nevertheless give rise to a series of neurophysiological disorders. Changes may also result from inflammation (encephalitis) caused by the immune activation induced by parasitization, which would increase inflammatory cytokines in the rodent brain, such as tumor necrosis factor alpha (TNF-α), interleukin-1β (IL-1β), IL-10, interferon gamma (IFNγ), C-reactive protein, tissue inhibitor of metalloproteinases 1 (TIMP-1), or vascular cell adhesion molecule 1 (VCAM-1), similar to observations in *postmortem* biopsies of schizophrenic patients. Finally, the behavioral changes have also been related to neurochemical mechanisms, with an increase in dopamine and homovanillic acid and a decrease in norepinephrine levels [73, 84, 85, 87–90].

Any of the above mechanisms in rodents could also produce behavioral changes in the brains of other intermediate hosts, including humans. Thus, research in humans also suggests that toxoplasmosis may alter behavior, psychomotor abilities, or personality, with the corresponding clinical consequences [84]. These disorders would be more related to latent rather than acute toxoplasmosis, given that its emergence, frequently several years after primary infection and not during the acute phase, would indicate that it results from slow and possibly accumulative changes induced by parasite activity [91–93]. The study by Horacek et al. [76] demonstrates that, in seropositive schizophrenic patients, latent parasitization is associated with a significant reduction in gray matter volume in specific brain areas (cortical regions, hippocampus, and caudate nucleus), which is not observed in seronegative patients.

Reinforcing the relationship between the parasite and the psychiatric disease, it has been demonstrated that haloperidol, an antipsychotic drug that blocks D2 dopaminergic receptors in the mesolimbic system and often used in the symptomatic treatment of schizophrenia, inhibits the replication of tachyzoites in cell cultures *in vitro*. This effect may at least partly be due to the capacity of this drug to inhibit calcium transport, blocking cell ion channels [94]. The interaction between tachyzoites and host cells is calcium-dependent; hence, cell invasion capacity can be inhibited by the presence of drugs that block calcium channels, such as haloperidol [95]. Experimental studies with rodents have also demonstrated that some behavioral changes caused by the infection are reverted by using the antipsychotic, and that there are fewer parasitized neurons and glial cells after the treatment; this is observed using immunohistochemical techniques [96]. It is therefore possible that its therapeutic effect can be explained in patients with schizophrenia by various mechanisms, given that on the one hand, it blocks dopamine, whose levels are often elevated in schizophrenia patients parasitized with *T. gondii* [89, 97], and on the other hand, it can inhibit parasite replication in brain cells [96]. Other antipsychotic drugs such as fluphenazine, thioridazine, trifluoperazine, or zuclopenthixol, and mood stabilizers, e.g., valproic acid, were also found to inhibit *T. gondii* proliferation in cell cultures [94, 98, 99].

Antipsychotics are especially indicated in patients with a predominance of positive symptoms and agitation (as in the acute phase of schizophrenia), which are significantly more frequent in those parasitized with *T. gondii*, as noted above. The greater effectiveness of these drugs in these situations may be due not only to their dopamine blocking effect but also to their anti-*Toxoplasma* activity. Thus, these treatments were found to reduce anti-*Toxoplasma* antibody levels in seropositive schizophrenic patients, indicating their antiparasitic effect [44]. These findings suggest that these drugs may possibly have a beneficial effect on schizophrenic patients parasitized with *T. gondii*.

Studies to date on the possible effect in these patients of drugs with anti-*Toxoplasma* activity (e.g., pyrimethamine, sulfadiazine, azithromycin, or trimethoprim-sulfamethoxazole) have not demonstrated significant improvements in psychotic symptoms [100, 101]. In fact, drugs used to treat toxoplasmosis are largely active during the tachyzoite replication phase, and their effectiveness against bradyzoites in tissue cysts is drastically reduced once chronic infection by *T. gondii* is established [102].

The etiological relationship between parasitization and schizophrenia has not yet been established, despite the above data on behavioral changes in animals or humans and on the effects of antipsychotic drugs on symptoms. In addition, differences in behavioral disorders between humans and rodents may mean that results in animal models cannot be extrapolated to humans. It should also be borne in mind that the mild behavioral modifications associated with the infection cannot necessarily be considered symptoms of a psychotic disease.

7. The role of proinflammatory cytokines

The host response to the parasitization of glial cells and neurons involves the activation of immune system cells, including T lymphocytes (CD4+ and CD8+), B lymphocytes, NK cells, macrophages, and dendritic and glial cells. These produce a wide variety of inflammatory cytokines such as IFNγ, interleukins (IL-1, IL-1β, IL-2, IL-4, IL-6, IL-10, IL-12, IL-15, IL-17, IL-18, IL-23), granulocyte macrophage colony-stimulating factor (GM-CSF), and/or TNFα [69, 103]. These cytokines halt protozoan proliferation and limit their replication, playing a key role in regulating the infection of host cells, thereby favoring the formation of tissue cysts and the development of the chronic latent form [20]. These and other inflammatory responses have also been reported in schizophrenia [104] and are therefore involved in brain disorders both in this disease and in *T. gondii* infection [105].

Thus, infection of brain tissue by *T. gondii* produces activation of the Jak/STAT pathway, which is recognized as an important regulatory mechanism in CNS development, function, and disease progression [106, 107]. This pathway comprises three elements: a ligand receptor, the majority are receptors of cytokines such as IFNγ; Janus kinase (Jak) proteins associated with the receptor within the cell, which possess tyrosine-kinase activity; and signal transducer and activator of transcription (STAT) proteins, which act as transcription factors that move toward the cell nucleus after their phosphorylation, where they bind with regulatory sequences of genes designated gamma interferon activation sites (GAS) [108]. In mammals, the Jak/STAT pathway induces the transcription of genes that participate in multiple processes, including antimicrobial activity and the production of proinflammatory cytokines [109]. Among other effects, an increase is produced in the expression of NADPH oxidase enzyme (NOX2) and inducible nitric oxide synthase (iNOS). These enzymes are responsible for the production of reactive oxygen species (ROS) and reactive nitrogen species (RNS), which assist the destruction of foreign pathogens [110, 111] but have been linked to seizures, stroke, neurodegenerative diseases, and schizophrenia [111, 112] as a consequence of their toxic effect on neurons [113]. Scientific evidence points to ROS-mediated oxidative damage as a key pathogenic pathway involved in infection-mediated neuropathy. According to these findings, it can be expected that a high degree of degenerated neuron degeneration and cognitive impairment is associated with the presence of *T. gondii* in the brain [111].

8. The importance of dopamine and other neurotransmitters

As already noted, some experimental animal and human studies concluded that behavioral changes may be explained by increased dopamine levels in the parasitized brain, and that these disorders could largely be resolved by administration of a dopaminergic receptor antagonist (e.g., haloperidol) or dopamine reuptake inhibitor (e.g., GBR-12909) [96, 114, 115]. It is therefore possible that dopamine represents the link between toxoplasmosis and schizophrenia [97]. This neurotransmitter is synthesized in the cytosol of neurons from L-tyrosine amino acid by the action of the tyrosine hydroxylase enzyme, which converts it to L-3,4-dihydroxyphenylalanine (L-DOPA). L-DOPA is in turn converted by the action of DOPA-decarboxylase (DDC) to dopamine, a precursor of norepinephrine (noradrenalin) and epinephrine (adrenalin) in the synthesis pathway of these catecholamines. It is subsequently packaged in vesicles and transported through the axon to the synapse, where it is released by exocytosis in response to an electrical stimulus. Dopamine is one of the main neurotransmitters in the prefrontal cortex and the mesolimbic system (mainly formed by the nucleus accumbens, amygdala, and hippocampus), where the presence of *T. gondii* tissue cysts is especially frequent [73].

The definitive mechanism by which *T. gondii* induces changes in the dopaminergic pathway has not been fully elucidated. However, an increase in dopamine with no modification of cellular tyrosine hydroxylase was demonstrated *in vitro* after parasitization of a rat pheochromocytoma cell line (PC12) and *in vivo* after the parasitization of mouse brains. This dopamine synthesis is attributable to the additional activity of the aromatic amino acid hydroxylase, which is encoded by two *T. gondii* genes [116] and has homologous activities to those of mammalian tyrosine hydroxylase, associated with the entry of cellular DDC enzymes into parasitophorous vacuoles (compartments formed by the parasite to invade the cell) and into tissue cysts (the protozoan encodes no enzyme with DDC activity) [114, 117]. Experiments in cell cultures have demonstrated that dopamine increases the replication of *T. gondii* tachyzoites [118]. This biochemical mechanism may play a role in the behavioral changes observed, which would result from the involvement of catecholaminergic neurons and consequent dopaminergic hyperactivity [19].

Parasitization in the fetal period may also impair the development of mesolimbic dopaminergic or prefrontal cortex neurons (inappropriate migration, altered position, reduced synapses, etc.) leading to neurodevelopmental disorders. Disease symptoms would not be induced immediately by these early anomalies but would rather manifest after a latency period of one to three decades. This is because the proliferation, migration, differentiation, and maturation of glial progenitor cells continue throughout childhood [119] and the volume of gray matter increases to a peak in puberty before beginning to diminish [120].

However, the hypothesis that increased dopamine levels or dopaminergic hyperactivity is the underlying cause of schizophrenia does not account for the negative symptoms in these patients, which are more likely to result from dopaminergic hypoactivity. Therefore, neurotransmitters other than dopamine may play an important role in the development of this disease. Thus, it has been proposed that deficits in glutamatergic brain systems also participate in the physiopathology of schizophrenia based on findings of higher kynurenic acid levels in patients with psychotic symptoms than in healthy controls [121]. Kynurenic acid is a metabolite of tryptophan with important biological effects on the nervous system, related to its antagonism for the glutamate receptor in the human brain (it is a glutamatergic NMDA receptor antagonist). Increased kynurenic acid levels due to blockade of NMDA receptors in glutamatergic neurons have been related to changes in dopamine level in different brain areas. These modifications include cortical dopaminergic hypoactivity and mesolimbic dopaminergic hyperactivity, which would explain the negative and positive symptoms in patients. This relationship between glutamate pathway disorders and dopamine level changes may explain the presence of different symptoms in the psychosis [122].

Indoleamine-2,3-dioxygenase and therefore the metabolism of tryptophan, a precursor metabolite in serotonin (and melatonin) synthesis, are induced by the proinflammatory cytokines released in response to *T. gondii* infection, especially IFNγ [123]. Tryptophan is an essential amino acid for the parasite, and decreased levels inhibit its growth and replication capacity [124]. However, induction of this metabolite in turn increases kynurenic acid levels and therefore alters dopamine levels through the glutamatergic receptor antagonist effect of this acid [114]. Tryptophan degradation also reduces serotonin levels, which has been related to a higher incidence of depression and suicide [125, 126], as also observed in patients with high anti-*T. gondii* antibody levels [56].

Patients with schizophrenia also show anomalous levels of gamma-aminobutyric acid (GABA), another important neurotransmitter [20], which is synthesized from glutamate by the action of glutamic acid decarboxylase (GAD) [127]. GABA activates $GABA_A$ receptors, which are ion channels, and $GABA_B$ receptors, which are G-protein-coupled receptors [128]. It is the main neurotransmitter with inhibiting effect in the CNS, regulating dopaminergic activity and playing a key role in the reduction of neuronal excitability throughout the nervous system. Dopaminergic neurons in basal ganglia would be directly inhibited by GABAergic neurons, so that any GABAergic hypofunction would be accompanied by an increase in subcortical dopaminergic activity, as observed in schizophrenia.

More direct evidence of the involvement of this neurotransmitter in the etiology of schizophrenia derives from data on the reduction in neurons in the GABAergic system or in brain regions such as the hippocampus, temporal lobe, and prefrontal cortex of schizophrenic patients [129–131]. *Postmortem* molecular studies have demonstrated: a reduction in messenger RNA (mRNA) levels of isoform 67 of glutamic acid decarboxylase (GAD67) and of type 1 GABA transporter (GAT-1) in the prefrontal cortex of schizophrenics [132, 133]; an increase in subunit $\alpha 2$ of the $GABA_A$ receptor in the initial segment of the axon of pyramidal neurons [134]; and a reduced expression of the receptor $GABA_{B,}$ which regulates GABA release as a possible compensatory mechanism for GABAergic dysfunction [135]. As noted above, these findings may be the consequence of alterations during neurodevelopment in the differentiation and migration of these neurons toward their definitive localizations in the brain. This would give rise to structural alterations and neurochemical dysregulation that would have a global effect on all of these neurotransmitters (dopamine, glutamate, serotonin, GABA) and would become manifest from adolescence onward, inducing the appearance of the disease. Once more, infection by *T. gondii* may play an important role in this process.

Outside the nervous system, GABAergic mechanisms have been observed in different tissues and peripheral organs, and GABA has also been found to exert a major role in the immune system, with important inter-regulatory functions between this and the CNS [136]. It has been reported that *T. gondii* infection is followed by an increase in the motility and migratory capacity of infected dendritic cells, permitting propagation of the parasite to different tissues, including the brain [128]. Although dendritic cells are considered guardians of the immune system, they can also, paradoxically, mediate in the spread of the parasite. This mechanism is produced by the induction in these cells of the GAD enzyme and therefore of GABA production and secretion, which in turn activate GABA receptors expressed by these same cells, stimulating their motility [137]. In experimental mouse models, inhibition of the GABAergic pathway by blockade of GABAA receptors or inhibition of the GAD enzyme markedly reduced the hypermotility and spread of *T. gondii*-infected dendritic cells and therefore of the parasite itself [137, 138]. Finally, it has also been reported that brain infection by *T. gondii* can interfere with the GABAergic system by inducing changes in the distribution of the GAD67 enzyme, although this event has been related more to possible neurological complications of toxoplasmic encephalitis, such as seizures [139], than to possible complications of latent toxoplasmosis, such as schizophrenia.

Accordingly, the inflammatory response of the host to parasitization, which aims to control parasite replication and alterations in differentiation and migration processes, can change levels of dopamine, tryptophan, kynurenic acid, serotonin, and GABA, leading to behavioral changes and giving rise to different psychotic symptoms.

In order to establish dopamine and other related neurotransmitters as a causal link between toxoplasmosis and schizophrenia development, it is necessary to confirm that this neurotransmitter is also involved in the disease genesis when there is infection by other pathogens [140], and this mechanism should also explain the possible contribution of *T. gondii* parasitization in other dopaminergic pathway diseases, e.g., Parkinson's disease [114].

9. The *N*-methyl-D-aspartate receptor hypofunction theory: anti-NMDAr antibodies

Encephalitis due to antibodies against the glutamatergic NMDA receptor (anti-NMDAr antibodies) is an autoimmune disease caused when antibodies produced by the host immune system identify NMDA receptors as foreign antigens. This receptor forms a heterotetramer between two GluN1 and two GluN2 subunits and participates in essential functions for reality perception, memory, and the control of unconscious activities. The disease is characterized by the hypofunction of NMDA receptors, which would account for the psychotic symptoms, personality changes, memory impairment, and psychomotor agitation

[141, 142]. It usually arises during the course of a paraneoplastic process and is frequently associated with the development of ovarian teratomas, explaining its higher incidence among females [143, 144]. Likewise, 14–75% of patients with systemic erythematous lupus, another autoimmune disease, have been reported to manifest psychiatric symptoms related to the presence of the same antibodies [145, 146]. This involvement of anti-NMDAr antibodies (and other neurotransmission receptors) indicates an important link between immune abnormalities and altered neurotransmission in schizophrenia, major depression, or bipolar disorder [147, 148].

The presence of anti-NMDAr antibodies has been documented in schizophrenic patients in the absence of seizures, movement disorders, or other neurological signs or symptoms [149–151], although other researchers were unable to replicate these findings [152, 153]. For various reasons, the production of anti-NMDAr antibodies is a plausible mechanism to explain at least a percentage of schizophrenic cases [149]: several studies reported that 5–10% of cases are associated with the presence of these antibodies in serum and cerebrospinal fluid [150, 151, 154]; kynurenic acid is an antagonist of glutamate *via* blockade of NMDA receptors, as commented in the previous section, suggesting that it contributes to the pathogenesis of schizophrenia [122]; persistent blockade of NMDA receptors in experimental animals recreates clinical characteristics of schizophrenia [155]; selective elimination of subunit GluN1 of the NMDA receptor in neurons of the cortex and hippocampus in early postnatal development contributes to the pathophysiology of schizophrenia-related disorders in mice [156]; some of the genes associated with schizophrenia are related to the NMDA receptor [157]; NMDA receptors are reduced in medication-free schizophrenic patients [158]; blockade of the receptor with ketamine or phencyclidine produces psychotic symptoms [159, 160]; and *de novo* mutations (large chromosomal copy number changes) affect genes that encode one or more nucleotides among the glutamatergic postsynaptic proteins that form part of the receptor, providing insight into possible etiological mechanisms underlying schizophrenia [161].

Maternal infection during brain development or infection during childhood may produce anti-NMDAr antibodies, while other environmental or genetic factors may influence the age of disease onset [149]. Certain pathogens have been associated with elevated anti-NMDAr antibodies [162, 163]. Thus, a *T. gondii*-infected mouse model showed a significantly higher increase in serum GluN2A autoantibodies among juvenile- *versus* adult-infected mice. Adolescence is a critical window in neurodevelopment, and the authors hypothesized that early infection would have greater effects on behavior and the brain in comparison with adult infection. It is possible that chronic infection with *T. gondii* affects pre- or postnatal brain development by altering synaptic maturation. An increase in NMDAr autoantibodies due to *T. gondii* exposure might underlie behavioral alterations in symptomatic individuals [164].

10. Studies on gene-infection interaction

Various studies have demonstrated the participation of numerous genes in schizophrenia, providing firm evidence on the involvement of genetics in the etiology of the disease

[165]. Some authors have described inheritability in >80% of cases, and schizophrenia has been associated with polymorphic variability in certain genes [21, 166–168]. However, the genetic hypothesis alone cannot explain the familial association of schizophrenia with other diseases, the seasonal peaks of schizophrenia births, the different prevalences among residents of urban and rural areas, discordant results between monozygotic and dizygotic twins or between dizygotic twins and full siblings, or correlations in adopted children, which are, however, consistent with an infectious etiology [1]. Schizophrenia is likely a genetically complex disease that does not follow a Mendelian transmission pattern but rather involves multiple genes, each with a small effect, which act in combination with epigenetic and environmental factors [169]. Accordingly, epidemiological findings suggest that a combination of intrinsic (genetic) and extrinsic or environmental factors, including infections, may participate in the origin of this disease, operating during the development of the individual at some time between conception and adolescence [7]. Tomonaga [170] proposed that persistent chronic infections or the expression of microbial proteins may directly and/or indirectly affect CNS functions in infected individuals, changing the expressions of genes related to schizophrenia and increasing the risk of suffering this disease or at least some of its varied clinical phenotypes.

Genes whose variants or polymorphisms have been associated with the risk of schizophrenia include some that encode proteins with important functions in neurodevelopment or neurodegeneration and in neuronal neurotransmission circuits. This is the case of the gene that encodes neuregulin 1 (NRG1), a key molecule in maintaining brain synaptic plasticity in adults, which has been related to schizophrenia etiology [171, 172], and the genes that encode catechol-O-methyltransferase (COMT) [173], proline dehydrogenase (PRODH) [174], dysbindin protein (DTNBP1) [175], a regulator of G4 protein (RGS4) [176], a regulator of potassium calcium channels (KCNN3) [177], and D-amino-oxidase complex (G72, DAAO) [178], among others [179]. The genes that encode these proteins are located in chromosomal regions that have been described as relevant for the study of schizophrenia, and many of these proteins participate in glutamatergic, dopaminergic, or serotonergic neurotransmission circuits.

Genetic polymorphisms that increase susceptibility to schizophrenia, including some of the above, have also been related to resistance or susceptibility to certain infections through their important role in the life cycle of some pathogens, including *T. gondii* [169, 179, 180]. Schizophrenia may possibly correspond to a model in which various genes may interact with microbial agents in a process that is probably mediated by the inflammatory and immune response of the individual, increasing the risk of developing psychiatric disease [169, 179–182]. It appears reasonable to assume that infections may interact, thereby changing the expressions of schizophrenia-related genes and increasing the risk of suffering this condition.

Various rodent [79, 183, 184] and human [185, 186] studies have supported the existence of genetic susceptibility to *T. gondii* parasitization, suggesting that if the parasite were one of the possible causes underlying schizophrenia development, this genetic susceptibility might also explain familial cases of schizophrenia [1]. As commented above, some *T. gondii* genes encode proteins with a similar activity to that of enzymes (e.g., tyrosine hydroxylase) in the cells of their intermediate hosts. Therefore, this parasite has genes that allow it to "manipulate" the behavior of the host and facilitate its capture by the cat, its definitive host, thereby favoring parasite survival. The presence of these genes is consequently an evolutionary advantage of *T. gondii* [19].

Genetic studies (in animals and humans) currently center on the possible presence of genes or specific allelic variants that interact with the genes of microorganisms that can infect the patient (gene-infection interaction hypothesis), increasing the risk of schizophrenia [187–189]. Thus, it has been demonstrated that a critical role in human congenital *T. gondii* infection is played by the *ALOX12* gene, which encodes arachidonate 5-lipoxygenase enzyme, which is involved in fatty acid metabolism and has been related to schizophrenia, at least in a Korean population [190, 191]. HLA-related genes such as *SGK1* on chromosome 6, which plays a role in regulating different brain functions [192] and mediates the effects of cortisol on hippocampal neurogenesis [193], have a modulating effect on some infectious agents, including *T. gondii*, consistent with the proposition that parasitization may modify the risk of schizophrenia [187]. In a study of mice parasitized with *T. gondii*, heterozygous deletion of the *Nurr1* gene (Nurr1 ± genotype), an orphan nuclear receptor essential for the development of mesencephalic dopamine neurons [194], predisposed the animals to behavioral disorders that involve dopamine neurotransmission associated with schizophrenia symptoms [195].

A further example in support of this hypothesis is the Akt cell signaling system. The *Akt* gene encodes a serine-threonine kinase with three isoforms (Akt1, 2, and 3), whose activation mediates cell survival processes and whose inhibition favors apoptosis. As commented above, the innate immune system induces a range of processes after infection of brain cells by *T. gondii*, including antimicrobial activity and the generation of ROS to assist in the destruction of foreign pathogens. However, increases in ROS concentrations activate the Akt system, which guarantees cell survival and allows the pathogen to persist and replicate within the infected cell. Akt is above all activated in pathophysiological situations in which ROS increase as the result of ischemia-reperfusion, playing an important role in the protection of the different cells and tissues involved, including nerve tissue [196]. On the other hand, Akt is known to affect dopaminergic signaling, and polymorphisms of the *Akt1* gene have been found to increase the risk of developing schizophrenia through its relationship with dopaminergic pathways of the prefrontal cortex [197].

Other researchers reported similar associations between schizophrenia risk and other human pathogens, supporting the gene-infection interaction hypothesis [198–201]. This research line on the effects of interaction between genes or genetic variants on the risk of schizophrenia related to *T. gondii* parasitization is highly likely to establish the true causes of the disease, at least in some types of patient.

11. Is there an etiological association between *Toxoplasma gondii* infection and schizophrenia development?

Numerous studies have contributed evidence on the involvement of toxoplasmosis in the pathogenesis of numerous CNS diseases, including bipolar disorder, depression, Alzheimer's disease, Parkinson's disease, and epilepsy [49, 202–204]. However, the main advances over the past few years have been achieved by research on deciphering the molecular mechanisms underlying the physiopathology of schizophrenia.

This chapter analyzes data from *in vitro* and animal and human *in vivo* studies in order elucidate points of connection between *T. gondii* and schizophrenia. It can be concluded that infection by *T. gondii* is highly likely to be a cause of the disease for the following reasons: it is a neurotropic microorganism that persistently invades glial cells and neurons; it generates brain development anomalies; it reduces brain gray matter density; it elicits an inflammatory and immune response that alters neurotransmission systems; it affects cognitive function and behavior; and its replication is inhibited by some antipsychotics. All disorders reported for the parasite are associated with the development of psychotic symptoms. Furthermore, specific genetic polymorphisms linked to an increased risk of schizophrenia have also been associated with a higher likelihood of infection by this parasite. Nevertheless, despite all of the above evidence on this possible pathogenic association, one important

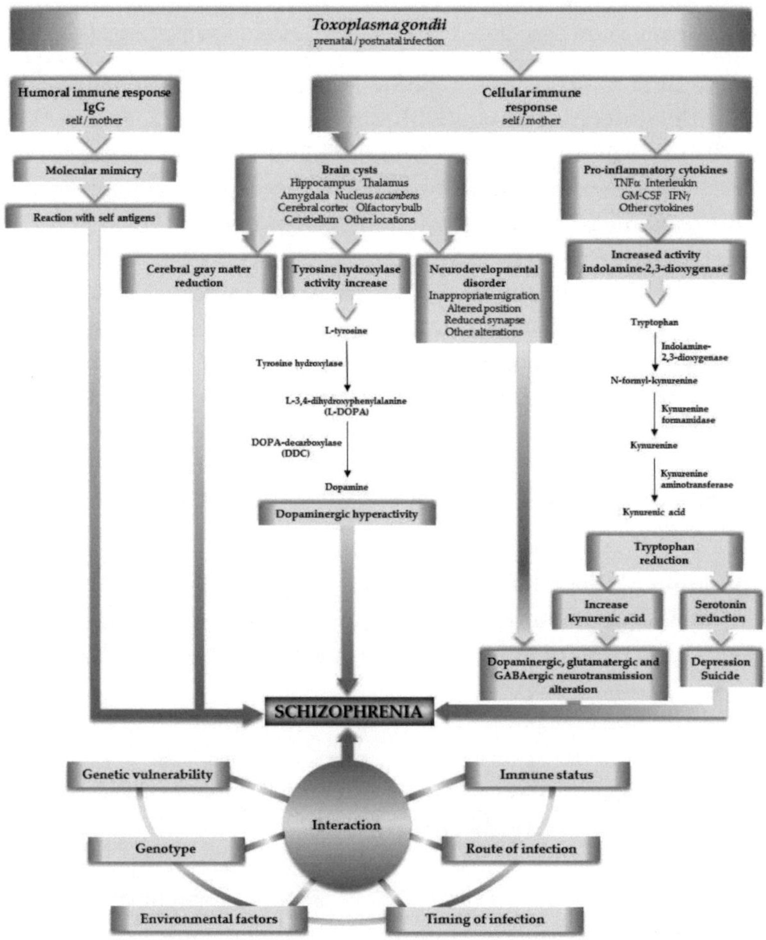

Figure 1. Likely involvement of infection by *Toxoplasma gondii* in the development of schizophrenia.

http://dx.doi.org/10.5772/66018

question remains to be resolved, which is why most individuals with signs of infection by *T. gondii* are asymptomatic and only a few develop psychiatric disorders.

Schizophrenia is a complex disease with innumerable symptoms, and its presentation and severity vary among patients. According to the infectious hypothesis of this disease (**Figure 1**), differences among patients would be influenced by their genetic predisposition or vulnerability, their immune status, the timing of parasitization (congenital, neonatal, or adult), the time interval since their first contact, and/or the particular brain area(s) affected. Characteristics of the infection also play a role, including its source (oocysts or tissue cysts), possible interactions with other infectious agents, and the genotype; thus, genotypes II and III more frequently establish chronic infections and show a greater expression of tyrosine hydroxylase genes in comparison with genotype I, and they may be more strongly related to behavioral changes [205].

Finally, the biology of schizophrenia must be fully elucidated to support the appropriate design of disease-modifying therapies or novel antipsychotic drugs. There appears to be sufficient evidence to suggest that schizophrenic patients with *T. gondii* infection could clinically benefit from a combined therapeutic approach based on the prescription of current or future antipsychotic drugs with antitoxoplasmic activity. However, published results have not been conclusive [206], and randomized controlled prospective trials are required in wider samples, stratifying schizophrenic patients into subgroups (e.g., by clinical phenotype, pathophysiological mechanism, or response to treatment) and in relation to specific types of *T. gondii* parasitization. Translational research must play a key role, with the involvement of psychiatric, neurologic, immunologic, biochemical, genetic, pharmacological, and microbiological investigators, among others, offering the possibility of using new and more effective methodologies. It appears highly likely that different causal agents are responsible for schizophrenia and that the pathogenic action of a particular microorganism such as *T. gondii* would only be relevant in certain patient subgroups, endorsing the need for personalized medicine.

Author details

Antonio Sorlozano-Puerto[1] and Jose Gutierrez-Fernandez[1,2]*

*Address all correspondence to: josegf@ugr.es

1 Department of Microbiology, School of Medicine, University of Granada and Biosanitary Research Institute ibs, Granada, Spain

2 Area of Microbiology, Granada University Hospital Complex, Spain

References

[1] Ledgerwood LG, Ewald PW, Cochran GM. Genes, germs, and schizophrenia: an evolutionary perspective. Perspect Biol Med. 2003;**46**(3):317–348. doi:10.1353/pbm.2003.0038

[2] Tsuang M. Schizophrenia: genes and environment. Biol Psychiatry. 2000;**47**(3):210–220. doi:10.1016/S0006-3223(99)00289-9

[3] Dinan TG, Borre YE, Cryan JF. Genomics of schizophrenia: time to consider the gut microbiome? Mol Psychiatry. 2014;**19**(12):1252–1257. doi:10.1038/mp.2014.93

[4] Arseneault L, Cannon M, Witton J, Murray RM. Causal association between cannabis and psychosis: examination of the evidence. Br J Psychiatry. 2004;**184**:110–117. doi:10.1192/bjp.184.2.110

[5] Brown AS. The risk for schizophrenia from childhood and adult infections. Am J Psychiatry. 2008;**165**(1):7–10. doi:10.1176/appi.ajp.2007.07101637

[6] Fatemi SH, Folsom TD. The neurodevelopmental hypothesis of schizophrenia, revisited. Schizophr Bull. 2009;**35**(3):528–548. doi:10.1093/schbul/sbn187

[7] Matheson SL, Shepherd AM, Carr VJ. How much do we know about schizophrenia and how well do we know it? Evidence from the Schizophrenia Library. Psychol Med. 2014;**44**(16):3387–3405. doi:10.1017/S0033291714000166

[8] Moore TH, Zammit S, Lingford-Hughes A, Barnes TR, Jones PB, Burke M, Lewis G. Cannabis use and risk of psychotic or affective mental health outcomes: a systematic review. Lancet. 2007;**370**(9584):319–328. doi:10.1016/S0140-6736(07)61162-3

[9] Sullivan PF, Kendler KS, Neale MC. Schizophrenia as a complex trait: evidence from a meta-analysis of twin studies. Arch Gen Psychiatry. 2003;**60**(12):1187–1192. doi:10.1001/archpsyc.60.12.1187

[10] Rawlins S. Nonviral sexually transmitted infections. J Obstet Gynecol Neonatal Nurs. 2001;**30**(3):324–331. doi:10.1111/j.1552-6909.2001.tb01551.x

[11] Arias I, Sorlozano A, Villegas E, de Dios Luna J, McKenney K, Cervilla J, Gutierrez B, Gutierrez J. Infectious agents associated with schizophrenia: a meta-analysis. Schizophr Res. 2012;**136**(1–3):128–136. doi:10.1016/j.schres.2011.10.026

[12] Müller N, Riedel M, Ackenheil M, Schwarz MJ. The role of immune function in schizophrenia: an overview. Eur Arch Psychiatry Clin Neurosci. 1999;**249**(Suppl 4):62–68. doi:10.1007/PL00014187

[13] Nahmias AJ, Nahmias SB, Danielsson D. The possible role of transplacentally acquired antibodies to infectious agents, with molecular mimicry to nervous system sialic acid epitopes, as causes of neuromental disorders: prevention and vaccine implications. Clin Dev Immunol. 2006;**13**(2–4):167–183. doi:10.1080/17402520600801745

[14] Gomez-Sintes R, Bortolozzi A, Artigas F, Lucas JJ. Reduced striatal dopamine DA D2 receptor function in dominant-negative GSK-3 transgenic mice. Eur Neuropsychopharmacol. 2014;**24**(9):1524–1533. doi:10.1016/j.euroneuro.2014.07.004

[15] Flegr J. Influence of latent *Toxoplasma* infection on human personality, physiology and morphology: pros and cons of the *Toxoplasma*-human model in studying the manipulation hypothesis. J Exp Biol. 2013;**216**(Pt 1):127–133. doi:10.1242/jeb.073635

[16] Gagne SS. Toxoplasmosis. Prim Care Update Ob Gyns. 2001;**8**(3):122–126. doi:10.1016/S1068-607X(00)00083-4

[17] Montoya JG, Liesenfeld O. Toxoplasmosis. Lancet. 2004;**363**(9425):1965–1976. doi:10.1016/S0140-6736(04)16412-X

[18] Bossi P, Caumes E, Paris L, Dardé ML, Bricaire F. *Toxoplasma gondii*-associated Guillain-Barré syndrome in an immunocompetent patient. J Clin Microbiol. 1998;**36**(12):3724–3725.

[19] McConkey GA, Martin HL, Bristow GC, Webster JP. *Toxoplasma gondii* infection and behaviour—location, location, location? J Exp Biol. 2013;**216**(Pt 1):113–119. doi:10.1242/jeb.074153.

[20] Fabiani S, Pinto B, Bruschi F. Toxoplasmosis and neuropsychiatric diseases: can serological studies establish a clear relationship? Neurol Sci. 2013;**34**(4):417–425. doi:10.1007/s10072-012-1197-4

[21] Jablensky AV, Kalaydjieva LV. Genetic epidemiology of schizophrenia: phenotypes, risk factors, and reproductive behavior. Am J Psychiatry. 2003;**160**(3):425–429. doi:10.1176/appi.ajp.160.3.425

[22] Johnson J, Suzuki Y, Mack D, Mui E, Estes R, David C, Skamene E, Forman J, McLeod R. Genetic analysis of influences on survival following *Toxoplasma gondii* infection. Int J Parasitol. 2002;**32**(2):179–185. doi:10.1016/S0020-7519(01)00321-6

[23] Bennedsen BE, Mortensen PB, Olesen AV, Henriksen TB. Congenital malformations, stillbirths, and infant deaths among children of women with schizophrenia. Arch Gen Psychiatry. 2001;**58**(7):674–679. doi:10.1001/archpsyc.58.7.674

[24] Sever JL, Ellenberg JH, Ley AC, Madden DL, Fuccillo DA, Tzan NR, Edmonds DM. Toxoplasmosis: maternal and pediatric findings in 23,000 pregnancies. Pediatrics. 1988;**82**(2):181–192.

[25] Torrey EF, Torrey BB, Burton-Bradley BG. The epidemiology of schizophrenia in Papua New Guinea. Am J Psychiatry. 1974;**131**(5):567–573.

[26] Wallace GD, Zigas V, Gajdusek DC. Toxoplasmosis and cats in New Guinea. Am J Trop Med Hyg. 1974;**23**(1):8–14.

[27] Ryan M, Hall SM, Barrett NJ, Balfour AH, Holliman RE, Joynson DH. Toxoplasmosis in England and Wales 1981 to 1992. Commun Dis Rep CDR Rev. 1995;**5**(2):R13–R21.

[28] Watt DC, Szulecka TK. The effect of sex, marriage and age at first admission on the hospitalization of schizophrenics during 2 years following discharge. Psychol Med. 1979;**9**(3):529–539. doi:10.1017/S0033291700032098

[29] Kruszon-Moran D, McQuillan GM. Seroprevalence of six infectious diseases among adults in the United States by race/ethnicity: data from the third national health and nutrition examination survey, 1988–94. Adv Data. 2005;**352**:1–9.

[30] Regier DA, Farmer ME, Rae DS, Myers JK, Kramer M, Robins LN, George LK, Karno M, Locke BZ. One-month prevalence of mental disorders in the United States and sociode-

mographic characteristics: the Epidemiologic Catchment Area study. Acta Psychiatr Scand. 1993;**88**(1):35–47. doi:10.1111/j.1600-0447.1993.tb03411.x

[31] Torrey EF, Yolken RH. *Toxoplasma gondii* and schizophrenia. Emerg Infect Dis. 2003;**9**(11):1375–1380.

[32] Gutiérrez-Fernández J, Luna Del Castillo J de D, Mañanes-González S, Carrillo-Ávila JA, Gutiérrez B, Cervilla JA, Sorlózano-Puerto A. Different presence of *Chlamydia pneumoniae*, herpes simplex virus type 1, human herpes virus 6, and *Toxoplasma gondii* in schizophrenia: meta-analysis and analytical study. Neuropsychiatr Dis Treat. 2015;**11**:843–852. doi:10.2147/NDT.S79285

[33] Torrey EF, Bartko JJ, Lun ZR, Yolken RH. Antibodies to *Toxoplasma gondii* in patients with schizophrenia: a meta-analysis. Schizophr Bull. 2007;**33**(3):729–736. doi:10.1093/schbul/sbl050

[34] Torrey EF, Bartko JJ, Yolken RH. *Toxoplasma gondii* and other risk factors for schizophrenia: an update. Schizophr Bull. 2012;**38**(3):642–647. doi:10.1093/schbul/sbs043

[35] Sutterland AL, Fond G, Kuin A, Koeter MW, Lutter R, van Gool T, Yolken R, Szoke A, Leboyer M, de Haan L. Beyond the association. *Toxoplasma gondii* in schizophrenia, bipolar disorder, and addiction: systematic review and meta-analysis. Acta Psychiatr Scand. 2015;**132**(3):161–179. doi:10.1111/acps.12423

[36] Dard C, Fricker-Hidalgo H, Brenier-Pinchart MP, Pelloux H. Relevance of and new developments in serology for toxoplasmosis. Trends Parasitol. 2016;**32**(6):492–506. doi:10.1016/j.pt.2016.04.001.

[37] Ahmad D, Mehdi S, Sayed HH, Sayed AK, Shirzad G. Serological survey of *Toxoplasma gondii* in schizophrenia patients referred to Psychiatric Hospital, Sari City, Iran. Trop Biomed. 2010;**27**(3):476–482.

[38] Alvarado-Esquivel C, Alanis-Quiñones OP, Arreola-Valenzuela MA, Rodríguez-Briones A, Piedra-Nevarez LJ, Duran-Morales E, Estrada-Martínez S, Martínez-García SA, Liesenfeld O. Seroepidemiology of *Toxoplasma gondii* infection in psychiatric inpatients in a northern Mexican city. BMC Infect Dis. 2006;**6**:178. doi:10.1186/1471-2334-6-178

[39] Alvarado-Esquivel C, Urbina-Álvarez JD, Estrada-Martínez S, Torres-Castorena A, Molotla-de-León G, Liesenfeld O, Dubey JP. *Toxoplasma gondii* infection and schizophrenia: a case control study in a low *Toxoplasma* seroprevalence Mexican population. Parasitol Int. 2011;**60**(2):151–155. doi:10.1016/j.parint.2010.12.003

[40] Amminger GP, McGorry PD, Berger GE, Wade D, Yung AR, Phillips LJ, Harrigan SM, Francey SM, Yolken RH. Antibodies to infectious agents in individuals at ultra-high risk for psychosis. Biol Psychiatry. 2007;**61**(10):1215–1217. doi:10.1016/j.biopsych.2006.09.034

[41] Cetinkaya Z, Yazar S, Gecici O, Namli MN. Anti-*Toxoplasma gondii* antibodies in patients with schizophrenia—preliminary findings in a Turkish sample. Schizophr Bull. 2007;**33**(3):789–791. doi:10.1093/schbul/sbm021

[42] El-Sahn AA, Shatat HZ, Ghitany EM. Seropositivity of toxoplasmosis in patients with schizophrenia. J Egypt Public Health Assoc. 2005;**80**(5–6):509–524.

[43] Hamidinejat H, Ghorbanpoor M, Hosseini H, Alavi SM, Nabavi L, Jalali MH, Borojeni MP, Jafari H, Mohammadaligol S. *Toxoplasma gondii* infection in first-episode and inpatient individuals with schizophrenia. Int J Infect Dis. 2010;**14**(11):e978–e981. doi:10.1016/j.ijid.2010.05.018

[44] Leweke FM, Gerth CW, Koethe D, Klosterkötter J, Ruslanova I, Krivogorsky B, Torrey EF, Yolken RH. Antibodies to infectious agents in individuals with recent onset schizophrenia. Eur Arch Psychiatry Clin Neurosci. 2004;**254**(1):4–8. doi:10.1007/s00406-004-0481-6

[45] Niebuhr DW, Millikan AM, Cowan DN, Yolken R, Li Y, Weber NS. Selected infectious agents and risk of schizophrenia among US military personnel. Am J Psychiatry. 2008;**165**(1):99–106. doi:10.1176/appi.ajp.2007.06081254

[46] Omar A, Bakar OC, Adam NF, Osman H, Osman A, Suleiman AH, Manaf MR, Selamat MI. Seropositivity and serointensity of *Toxoplasma gondii* antibodies and DNA among patients with schizophrenia. Korean J Parasitol. 2015;**53**(1):29–34. doi:10.3347/kjp.2015.53.1.29

[47] Pedersen MG, Stevens H, Pedersen CB, Nørgaard-Pedersen B, Mortensen PB. *Toxoplasma* infection and later development of schizophrenia in mothers. Am J Psychiatry. 2011;**168**(8):814–821. doi:10.1176/appi.ajp.2011.10091351

[48] Tamer GS, Dundar D, Yalug I, Caliskan S, Yazar S, Aker A. The schizophrenia and *Toxoplasma gondii* connection: infectious, immune or both? Adv Ther. 2008;**25**(7):703–709. doi:10.1007/s12325-008-0063-5

[49] Tedla Y, Shibre T, Ali O, Tadele G, Woldeamanuel Y, Asrat D, Aseffa A, Mihret W, Abebe M, Alem A, Medhin G, Habte A. Serum antibodies to *Toxoplasma gondii* and *Herpesvidae* family viruses in individuals with schizophrenia and bipolar disorder: a case-control study. Ethiop Med J. 2011;**49**(3):211–220.

[50] Wang HL, Wang GH, Li QY, Shu C, Jiang MS, Guo Y. Prevalence of *Toxoplasma* infection in first-episode schizophrenia and comparison between *Toxoplasma*-seropositive and *Toxoplasma*-seronegative schizophrenia. Acta Psychiatr Scand. 2006;**114**(1):40–48. doi:10.1111/j.1600-0447.2006.00780.x

[51] Yolken RH, Bachmann S, Ruslanova I, Lillehoj E, Ford G, Torrey EF, Schroeder J. Antibodies to *Toxoplasma gondii* in individuals with first-episode schizophrenia. Clin Infect Dis. 2001;**32**(5):842–844. doi:10.1086/319221

[52] Xiao Y, Yin J, Jiang N, Xiang M, Hao L, Lu H, Sang H, Liu X, Xu H, Ankarklev J, Lindh J, Chen Q. Seroepidemiology of human *Toxoplasma gondii* infection in China. BMC Infect Dis. 2010;**10**:4. doi:10.1186/1471-2334-10-4.

[53] Nascimento FS, de Rosalmeida Dantas C, Netto MP, Mella LF, Suzuki LA, Banzato CE, Rossi CL. Prevalence of antibodies to *Toxoplasma gondii* in patients with schizophrenia and mood disorders. Schizophr Res. 2012;**142**(1–3):244–245. doi:10.1016/j.schres.2012.08.036

[54] Holub D, Flegr J, Dragomirecká E, Rodriguez M, Preiss M, Novák T, Čermák J, Horáček J, Kodym P, Libiger J, Höschl C, Motlová LB. Differences in onset of disease and severity of psychopathology between toxoplasmosis-related and toxoplasmosis-unrelated schizophrenia. Acta Psychiatr Scand. 2013;**127**(3):227–238. doi:10.1111/acps.12031

[55] Dickerson F, Boronow J, Stallings C, Origoni A, Yolken R. *Toxoplasma gondii* in individuals with schizophrenia: association with clinical and demographic factors and with mortality. Schizophr Bull. 2007;**33**(3):737–740. doi:10.1093/schbul/sbm005

[56] Okusaga O, Langenberg P, Sleemi A, Vaswani D, Giegling I, Hartmann AM, Konte B, Friedl M, Groer MW, Yolken RH, Rujescu D, Postolache TT. *Toxoplasma gondii* antibody titers and history of suicide attempts in patients with schizophrenia. Schizophr Res. 2011;**133**(1–3):150–155. doi:10.1016/j.schres.2011.08.006

[57] Rice JS, Kowal C, Volpe BT, DeGiorgio LA, Diamond B. Molecular mimicry: anti-DNA antibodies bind microbial and nonnucleic acid self-antigens. Curr Top Microbiol Immunol. 2005;**296**:137–151. doi:10.1007/3-540-30791-5_8

[58] Monroe JM, Buckley PF, Miller BJ. Meta-Analysis of anti-*Toxoplasma gondii* IgM antibodies in acute psychosis. Schizophr Bull. 2015;**41**(4):989–998. doi:10.1093/schbul/sbu159

[59] Mortensen PB, Nørgaard-Pedersen B, Waltoft BL, Sørensen TL, Hougaard D, Torrey EF, Yolken RH. *Toxoplasma gondii* as a risk factor for early-onset schizophrenia: analysis of filter paper blood samples obtained at birth. Biol Psychiatry. 2007;**61**(5):688–693. doi:10.1016/j.biopsych.2006.05.024

[60] Brown AS, Schaefer CA, Quesenberry CP Jr, Liu L, Babulas VP, Susser ES. Maternal exposure to toxoplasmosis and risk of schizophrenia in adult offspring. Am J Psychiatry. 2005;**162**(4):767–773. doi:10.1176/appi.ajp.162.4.767

[61] Blomström A, Karlsson H, Wicks S, Yang S, Yolken RH, Dalman C. Maternal antibodies to infectious agents and risk for non-affective psychoses in the offspring-a matched case-control study. Schizophr Res. 2012;**140**(1–3):25–30. doi:10.1016/j.schres.2012.06.035

[62] Buka SL, Tsuang MT, Torrey EF, Klebanoff MA, Wagner RL, Yolken RH. Maternal cytokine levels during pregnancy and adult psychosis. Brain Behav Immun. 2001;**15**(4):411–420. doi:10.1006/brbi.2001.0644

[63] Xiao J, Buka SL, Cannon TD, Suzuki Y, Viscidi RP, Torrey EF, Yolken RH. Serological pattern consistent with infection with type I *Toxoplasma gondii* in mothers and risk of psychosis among adult offspring. Microbes Infect. 2009;**11**(13):1011–1018. doi:10.1016/j.micinf.2009.07.007

[64] Mortensen PB, Nørgaard-Pedersen B, Waltoft BL, Sørensen TL, Hougaard D, Yolken RH. Early infections of *Toxoplasma gondii* and the later development of schizophrenia. Schizophr Bull. 2007;**33**(3):741–744. doi:10.1093/schbul/sbm009

[65] Lebech M, Andersen O, Christensen NC, Hertel J, Nielsen HE, Peitersen B, Rechnitzer C, Larsen SO, Nørgaard-Pedersen B, Petersen E. Feasibility of neonatal screening for toxoplasma infection in the absence of prenatal treatment. Danish Congenital Toxoplasmosis Study Group. Lancet. 1999;**353**(9167):1834–1837.

[66] Pope RM. Immunoregulatory mechanisms present in the maternal circulation during pregnancy. Baillieres Clin Rheumatol. 1990;**4**(1):33–52. doi:10.1016/S0950-3579(05)80242-0

[67] Brown AS, Hooton J, Schaefer CA, Zhang H, Petkova E, Babulas V, Perrin M, Gorman JM, Susser ES. Elevated maternal interleukin-8 levels and risk of schizophrenia in adult offspring. Am J Psychiatry. 2004;**161**(5):889–895. doi:10.1176/appi.ajp.161.5.889

[68] Buka SL, Tsuang MT, Torrey EF, Klebanoff MA, Bernstein D, Yolken RH. Maternal infections and subsequent psychosis among offspring. Arch Gen Psychiatry. 2001;**58**(11):1032–1037. doi:10.1001/archpsyc.58.11.1032

[69] Carruthers VB, Suzuki Y. Effects of *Toxoplasma gondii* infection on the brain. Schizophr Bull. 2007;**33**(3):745–751. doi:10.1093/schbul/sbm008

[70] Berenreiterová M, Flegr J, Kuběna AA, Němec P. The distribution of *Toxoplasma gondii* cysts in the brain of a mouse with latent toxoplasmosis: implications for the behavioral manipulation hypothesis. PLoS One. 2011;**6**(12):e28925. doi:10.1371/journal.pone.0028925

[71] Di Cristina M, Marocco D, Galizi R, Proietti C, Spaccapelo R, Crisanti A. Temporal and spatial distribution of *Toxoplasma gondii* differentiation into bradyzoites and tissue cyst formation *in vivo*. Infect Immun. 2008;**76**(8):3491–3501. doi:10.1128/IAI.00254-08

[72] Hermes G, Ajioka JW, Kelly KA, Mui E, Roberts F, Kasza K, Mayr T, Kirisits MJ, Wollmann R, Ferguson DJ, Roberts CW, Hwang JH, Trendler T, Kennan RP, Suzuki Y, Reardon C, Hickey WF, Chen L, McLeod R. Neurological and behavioral abnormalities, ventricular dilatation, altered cellular functions, inflammation, and neuronal injury in brains of mice due to common, persistent, parasitic infection. J Neuroinflamm. 2008;**5**:48. doi:10.1186/1742-2094-5-48

[73] Vyas A, Kim SK, Giacomini N, Boothroyd JC, Sapolsky RM. Behavioral changes induced by *Toxoplasma* infection of rodents are highly specific to aversion of cat odors. Proc Natl Acad Sci U S A. 2007;**104**(15):6442–6447. doi:10.1073/pnas.0608310104

[74] Cotter DR, Pariante CM, Everall IP. Glial cell abnormalities in major psychiatric disorders: the evidence and implications. Brain Res Bull. 2001;**55**(5):585–595. doi:10.1016/S0361-9230(01)00527-5

[75] Shenton ME, Dickey CC, Frumin M, McCarley RW. A review of MRI findings in schizophrenia. Schizophr Res. 2001;**49**(1–2):1–52. doi:10.1016/S0920-9964(01)00163-3

[76] Horacek J, Flegr J, Tintera J, Verebova K, Spaniel F, Novak T, Brunovsky M, Bubenikova-Valesova V, Holub D, Palenicek T, Höschl C. Latent toxoplasmosis reduces gray matter density in schizophrenia but not in controls: voxel-based-morphometry (VBM) study. World J Biol Psychiatry. 2012;**13**(7):501–509. doi:10.3109/15622975.2011.573809

[77] Conejero-Goldberg C, Torrey EF, Yolken RH. Herpesviruses and *Toxoplasma gondii* in orbital frontal cortex of psychiatric patients. Schizophr Res. 2003;**60**(1):65–69. doi:10.1016/S0920-9964(02)00160-3

[78] Berdoy M, Webster JP, Macdonald DW. Parasite-altered behaviour: is the effect of *Toxoplasma gondii* on *Rattus norvegicus* specific? Parasitology. 1995;**111**(Pt 4):403–409. doi:10.1017/S0031182000065902

[79] Berdoy M, Webster JP, Macdonald DW. Fatal attraction in rats infected with *Toxoplasma gondii*. Proc Biol Sci. 2000;**267**(1452):1591–1594. doi:10.1098/rspb.2000.1182

[80] Hay J, Aitken PP, Graham DI. Toxoplasma infection and response to novelty in mice. Z Parasitenkd. 1984;**70**(5):575–588. doi:10.1007/BF00926588

[81] Webster JP. The effect of *Toxoplasma gondii* and other parasites on activity levels in wild and hybrid *Rattus norvegicus*. Parasitology. 1994;**109**(Pt 5):583–589. doi:10.1017/S0031182000076460

[82] Webster JP, Brunton CF, MacDonald DW. Effect of *Toxoplasma gondii* upon neophobic behaviour in wild brown rats, *Rattus norvegicus*. Parasitology. 1994;**109**(Pt 1):37–43. doi:10.1017/S003118200007774X

[83] Witting PA. Learning capacity and memory of normal and *Toxoplasma*-infected laboratory rats and mice. Z Parasitenkd. 1979;**61**(1):29–51.

[84] Webster JP. Rats, cats, people and parasites: the impact of latent toxoplasmosis on behaviour. Microbes Infect. 2001;**3**(12):1037–1045. doi:10.1016/S1286-4579(01)01459-9

[85] Webster JP. The effect of *Toxoplasma gondii* on animal behavior: playing cat and mouse. Schizophr Bull. 2007;**33**(3):752–756. doi:10.1093/schbul/sbl073

[86] Hari Dass SA, Vyas A. *Toxoplasma gondii* infection reduces predator aversion in rats through epigenetic modulation in the host medial amygdala. Mol Ecol. 2014;**23**(24):6114–6122. doi:10.1111/mec.12888

[87] Daniels BP, Sestito SR, Rouse ST. An expanded task battery in the Morris water maze reveals effects of *Toxoplasma gondii* infection on learning and memory in rats. Parasitol Int. 2015;**64**(1):5–12. doi:10.1016/j.parint.2014.09.002

[88] Holliman RE. Toxoplasmosis, behaviour and personality. J Infect. 1997;**35**(2):105–110. doi:10.1016/S0163-4453(97)91380-3

[89] Stibbs HH. Changes in brain concentrations of catecholamines and indoleamines in *Toxoplasma gondii* infected mice. Ann Trop Med Parasitol. 1985;**79**(2):153–157.

[90] Tomasik J, Schultz TL, Kluge W, Yolken RH, Bahn S, Carruthers VB. Shared immune and repair markers during experimental *Toxoplasma* chronic brain infection and schizophrenia. Schizophr Bull. 2016;**42**(2):386–395. doi:10.1093/schbul/sbv134

[91] Flegr J, Zitková S, Kodym P, Frynta D. Induction of changes in human behaviour by the parasitic protozoan *Toxoplasma gondii*. Parasitology. 1996;**113**(Pt 1):49–54. doi:10.1017/S0031182000066269

[92] Flegr J, Kodym P, Tolarová V. Correlation of duration of latent *Toxoplasma gondii* infection with personality changes in women. Biol Psychol. 2000;**53**(1):57–68. doi:10.1016/S0301-0511(00)00034-X

[93] Havlícek J, Gasová ZG, Smith AP, Zvára K, Flegr J. Decrease of psychomotor performance in subjects with latent 'asymptomatic' toxoplasmosis. Parasitology. 2001;**122**(Pt 5):515–520. doi:10.1017/S0031182001007624

[94] Jones-Brando L, Torrey EF, Yolken R. Drugs used in the treatment of schizophrenia and bipolar disorder inhibit the replication of *Toxoplasma gondii*. Schizophr Res. 2003;**62**(3):237–244. doi:10.1016/S0920-9964(02)00357-2

[95] Pezzella N, Bouchot A, Bonhomme A, Pingret L, Klein C, Burlet H, Balossier G, Bonhomme P, Pinon JM. Involvement of calcium and calmodulin in *Toxoplasma gondii* tachyzoite invasion. Eur J Cell Biol. 1997;**74**(1):92–101.

[96] Webster JP, Lamberton PH, Donnelly CA, Torrey EF. Parasites as causative agents of human affective disorders? The impact of anti-psychotic, mood-stabilizer and anti-parasite medication on *Toxoplasma gondii*'s ability to alter host behaviour. Proc Biol Sci. 2006;**273**(1589):1023–1030. doi:10.1098/rspb.2005.3413

[97] Flegr J, Preiss M, Klose J, Havlícek J, Vitáková M, Kodym P. Decreased level of psychobiological factor novelty seeking and lower intelligence in men latently infected with the protozoan parasite *Toxoplasma gondii*. Dopamine, a missing link between schizophrenia and toxoplasmosis? Biol Psychol. 2003;**63**(3):253–268. doi:10.1016/S0301-0511(03)00075-9

[98] Fond G, Macgregor A, Tamouza R, Hamdani N, Meary A, Leboyer M, Dubremetz JF. Comparative analysis of anti-toxoplasmic activity of antipsychotic drugs and valproate. Eur Arch Psychiatry Clin Neurosci. 2014;**264**(2):179–183. doi:10.1007/s00406-013-0413-4

[99] Goodwin DG, Strobl JS, Lindsay DS. Evaluation of five antischizophrenic agents against *Toxoplasma gondii* in human cell cultures. J Parasitol. 2011;**97**(1):148–151. doi:10.1645/GE-2536.1

[100] Dickerson FB, Stallings CR, Boronow JJ, Origoni AE, Yolken RH. A double-blind trial of adjunctive azithromycin in individuals with schizophrenia who are seropositive for *Toxoplasma gondii*. Schizophr Res. 2009;**112**(1–3):198–199. doi:10.1016/j.schres.2009.05.005

[101] Shibre T, Alem A, Abdulahi A, Araya M, Beyero T, Medhin G, Deyassa N, Negash A, Nigatu A, Kebede D, Fekadu A. Trimethoprim as adjuvant treatment in schizophrenia: a double-blind, randomized, placebo-controlled clinical trial. Schizophr Bull. 2010;**36**(4):846–851. doi:10.1093/schbul/sbn191

[102] Wei HX, Wei SS, Lindsay DS, Peng HJ. A systematic review and meta-analysis of the efficacy of anti-*Toxoplasma gondii* medicines in humans. PLoS One. 2015;**10**(9):e0138204. doi:10.1371/journal.pone.0138204

[103] da Silva RC, Langoni H. *Toxoplasma gondii*: host-parasite interaction and behavior manipulation. Parasitol Res. 2009;**105**(4):893–898. doi:10.1007/s00436-009-1526-6

[104] Khandaker GM, Cousins L, Deakin J, Lennox BR, Yolken R, Jones PB. Inflammation and immunity in schizophrenia: implications for pathophysiology and treatment. Lancet Psychiatry. 2015;**2**(3):258–270. doi:10.1016/S2215-0366(14)00122-9

[105] Doorduin J, de Vries EF, Willemsen AT, de Groot JC, Dierckx RA, Klein HC. Neuroinflammation in schizophrenia-related psychosis: a PET study. J Nucl Med. 2009;**50**(11):1801–1807. doi:10.2967/jnumed.109.066647

[106] Lin G, Zhang H, Sun F, Lu Z, Reed-Maldonado A, Lee YC, Wang G, Banie L, Lue TF. Brain-derived neurotrophic factor promotes nerve regeneration by activating the JAK/STAT pathway in Schwann cells. Transl Androl Urol. 2016;**5**(2):167–175. doi:10.21037/tau.2016.02.03

[107] Qin H, Buckley JA, Li X, Liu Y, Fox TH 3rd, Meares GP, Yu H, Yan Z, Harms AS, Li Y, Standaert DG, Benveniste EN. Inhibition of the JAK/STAT pathway protects against α-synuclein-induced neuroinflammation and dopaminergic neurodegeneration. J Neurosci. 2016;**36**(18):5144–5159. doi:10.1523/JNEUROSCI.4658-15.2016

[108] Gavrilescu LC, Butcher BA, Del Rio L, Taylor GA, Denkers EY. STAT1 is essential for antimicrobial effector function but dispensable for gamma interferon production during *Toxoplasma gondii* infection. Infect Immun. 2004;**72**(3):1257–1264. doi:10.1128/IAI.72.3.1257-1264.2004

[109] Kim SK, Fouts AE, Boothroyd JC. *Toxoplasma gondii* dysregulates IFN-gamma-inducible gene expression in human fibroblasts: insights from a genome-wide transcriptional profiling. J Immunol. 2007;**178**(8):5154–5165.

[110] Sun GY, Horrocks LA, Farooqui AA. The roles of NADPH oxidase and phospholipases A2 in oxidative and inflammatory responses in neurodegenerative diseases. J Neurochem. 2007;**103**(1):1–16.

[111] Elsheikha HM, Büsselberg D, Zhu XQ. The known and missing links between *Toxoplasma gondii* and schizophrenia. Metab Brain Dis. 2016;**31**(4):749–759. doi:10.1007/s11011-016-9822-1

[112] Vasconcelos AR, Yshii LM, Viel TA, Buck HS, Mattson MP, Scavone C, Kawamoto EM. Intermittent fasting attenuates lipopolysaccharide-induced neuroinflammation and memory impairment. J Neuroinflamm. 2014;**11**:85. doi:10.1186/1742-2094-11-85

[113] Zindler E, Zipp F. Neuronal injury in chronic CNS inflammation. Best Pract Res Clin Anaesthesiol. 2010;**24**(4):551–562. doi:10.1016/j.bpa.2010.11.001

[114] Prandovszky E, Gaskell E, Martin H, Dubey JP, Webster JP, McConkey GA. The neurotropic parasite *Toxoplasma gondii* increases dopamine metabolism. PLoS One. 2011;**6**(9):e232866. doi:10.1371/journal.pone.0023866

[115] Skallová A, Kodym P, Frynta D, Flegr J. The role of dopamine in *Toxoplasma*-induced behavioural alterations in mice: an ethological and ethopharmacological study. Parasitology. 2006;**133**(Pt 5):525–535. doi:10.1017/S0031182006000886

[116] Gaskell EA, Smith JE, Pinney JW, Westhead DR, McConkey GA. A unique dual activity amino acid hydroxylase in *Toxoplasma gondii*. PLoS One. 2009;**4**(3):e4801. doi:10.1371/journal.pone.0004801

[117] Martin HL, Alsaady I, Howell G, Prandovszky E, Peers C, Robinson P, McConkey GA. Effect of parasitic infection on dopamine biosynthesis in dopaminergic cells. Neuroscience. 2015;**306**:50–62. doi:10.1016/j.neuroscience.2015.08.005

[118] Strobl JS, Goodwin DG, Rzigalinski BA, Lindsay DS. Dopamine stimulates propagation of *Toxoplasma gondii* tachyzoites in human fibroblast and primary neonatal rat astrocyte cell cultures. J Parasitol. 2012;**98**(6):1296–1299. doi:10.1645/GE-2760.1

[119] Stiles J, Jernigan TL. The basics of brain development. Neuropsychol Rev. 2010;**20**(4):327–348. doi:10.1007/s11065-010-9148-4

[120] Paus T. Mapping brain maturation and cognitive development during adolescence. Trends Cogn Sci. 2005;**9**(2):60–88. doi:10.1016/j.tics.2004.12.008

[121] Nilsson LK, Linderholm KR, Engberg G, Paulson L, Blennow K, Lindström LH, Nordin C, Karanti A, Persson P, Erhardt S. Elevated levels of kynurenic acid in the cerebrospinal fluid of male patients with schizophrenia. Schizophr Res. 2005;**80**(2–3):315–322. doi:10.1016/j.schres.2005.07.013

[122] Erhardt S, Schwieler L, Nilsson L, Linderholm K, Engberg G. The kynurenic acid hypothesis of schizophrenia. Physiol Behav. 2007;**92**(1–2):203–209. doi:10.1016/j.physbeh.2007.05.025

[123] Silva NM, Rodrigues CV, Santoro MM, Reis LF, Alvarez-Leite JI, Gazzinelli RT. Expression of indoleamine 2,3-dioxygenase, tryptophan degradation, and kynurenine formation during *in vivo* infection with *Toxoplasma gondii*: induction by endogenous gamma interferon and requirement of interferon regulatory factor 1. Infect Immun. 2002;**70**(2):859–868. doi:10.1128/IAI.70.2.859-868.2002

[124] Miller CM, Boulter NR, Ikin RJ, Smith NC. The immunobiology of the innate response to *Toxoplasma gondii*. Int J Parasitol. 2009;**39**(1):23–39. doi:10.1016/j.ijpara.2008.08.002

[125] Lidberg L, Belfrage H, Bertilsson L, Evenden MM, Asberg M. Suicide attempts and impulse control disorder are related to low cerebrospinal fluid 5-HIAA in mentally disordered violent offenders. Acta Psychiatr Scand. 2000;**101**(5):395–402.

[126] Widner B, Laich A, Sperner-Unterweger B, Ledochowski M, Fuchs D. Neopterin production, tryptophan degradation, and mental depression—what is the link? Brain Behav Immun. 2002;**16**(5):590–595. doi:10.1016/S0889-1591(02)00006-5

[127] Buddhala C, Hsu CC, Wu JY. A novel mechanism for GABA synthesis and packaging into synaptic vesicles. Neurochem Int. 2009;**55**(1–3):9–12. doi:10.1016/j.neuint.2009.01.020

[128] Barragan A, Weidner JM, Jin Z, Korpi ER, Birnir B. GABAergic signalling in the immune system. Acta Physiol (Oxf). 2015;**213**(4):819–827. doi:10.1111/apha.12467

[129] Simpson MD, Slater P, Deakin JF, Royston MC, Skan WJ. Reduced GABA uptake sites in the temporal lobe in schizophrenia. Neurosci Lett. 1989;**107**(1–3):211–215. doi:10.1016/0304-3940(89)90819-7

[130] Reynolds GP, Czudek C, Andrews HB. Deficit and hemispheric asymmetry of GABA uptake sites in the hippocampus in schizophrenia. Biol Psychiatry 1990;**27**(9):1038–1044. doi:10.1016/0006-3223(90)90039-5

[131] Lewis DA, Pierri JN, Volk DW, Melchitzky DS, Woo TU. Altered GABA neurotransmission and prefrontal cortical dysfunction in schizophrenia. Biol Psychiatry. 1999; **46**(5):616–626. doi:10.1016/S0006-3223(99)00061-X

[132] Volk D, Austin M, Pierri J, Sampson A, Lewis D. GABA transporter-1 mRNA in the prefrontal cortex in schizophrenia: decreased expression in a subset of neurons. Am J Psychiatry. 2001;**158**(2):256–265. doi:10.1176/appi.ajp.158.2.256

[133] Woo TU, Walsh JP, Benes FM. Density of glutamic acid decarboxylase 67 messenger RNA-containing neurons that express the *N*-methyl-D-aspartate receptor subunit NR2A in the anterior cingulate cortex in schizophrenia and bipolar disorder. Arch Gen Psychiatry. 2004;61(7):649–657.

[134] Volk DW, Pierri JN, Fritschy JM, Auh S, Sampson AR, Lewis DA. Reciprocal alterations in pre- and postsynaptic inhibitory markers at chandelier cell inputs to pyramidal neurons in schizophrenia. Cereb Cortex. 2002;**12**(10):1063–1070. doi:10.1093/cercor/12.10.1063

[135] Fatemi SH, Folsom TD, Thuras PD. Deficits in GABA(B) receptor system in schizophrenia and mood disorders: a postmortem study. Schizophr Res. 2011;**128**(1–3):37–43. doi:10.1016/j.schres.2010.12.025

[136] Olofsson PS, Rosas-Ballina M, Levine YA, Tracey KJ. Rethinking inflammation: neural circuits in the regulation of immunity. Immunol Rev. 2012;**248**(1):188–204. doi:10.1111/j.1600-065X.2012.01138.x

[137] Fuks JM, Arrighi RB, Weidner JM, Kumar Mendu S, Jin Z, Wallin RP, Rethi B, Birnir B, Barragan A. GABAergic signaling is linked to a hypermigratory phenotype in dendritic cells infected by *Toxoplasma gondii*. PLoS Pathog. 2012;**8**(12):e1003051. doi:10.1371/journal.ppat.1003051

[138] Weidner JM, Kanatani S, Hernandez-Castaneda MA, Fuks JM, Rethi B, Wallin RP, Barragan A. Rapid cytoskeleton remodelling in dendritic cells following invasion by *Toxoplasma gondii* coincides with the onset of a hypermigratory phenotype. Cell Microbiol. 2013;**15**(10):1735–1752. doi:10.1111/cmi.12145

[139] Brooks JM, Carrillo GL, Su J, Lindsay DS, Fox MA, Blader IJ. *Toxoplasma gondii* infections alter GABAergic synapses and signaling in the central nervous system. MBio. 2015;**6**(6):e01428–15. doi:10.1128/mBio.01428-15

[140] Xiao J, Li Y, Prandovszky E, Karuppagounder SS, Talbot CC Jr, Dawson VL, Dawson TM, Yolken RH. MicroRNA-132 dysregulation in *Toxoplasma gondii* infection has implications for dopamine signaling pathway. Neuroscience. 2014;**268**:128–138. doi:10.1016/j.neuroscience.2014.03.015

[141] Dalmau J, Gleichman AJ, Hughes EG, Rossi JE, Peng X, Lai M, Dessain SK, Rosenfeld MR, Balice-Gordon R, Lynch DR. Anti-NMDA-receptor encephalitis: case series and analysis of the effects of antibodies. Lancet Neurol. 2008;**7**(12):1091–1098. doi:10.1016/S1474-4422(08)70224-2

[142] Irani SR, Bera K, Waters P, Zuliani L, Maxwell S, Zandi MS, Friese MA, Galea I, Kullmann DM, Beeson D, Lang B, Bien CG, Vincent A. *N*-methyl-D-aspartate antibody encephalitis: temporal progression of clinical and paraclinical observations in a predominantly non-paraneoplastic disorder of both sexes. Brain. 2010;**133**(Pt 6):1655–1667. doi:10.1093/brain/awq113

[143] Dalmau J, Tüzün E, Wu HY, Masjuan J, Rossi JE, Voloschin A, Baehring JM, Shimazaki H, Koide R, King D, Mason W, Sansing LH, Dichter MA, Rosenfeld MR, Lynch DR. Paraneoplastic anti-*N*-methyl-D-aspartate receptor encephalitis associated with ovarian teratoma. Ann Neurol. 2007;**61**(1):25–36. doi:10.1002/ana.21050

[144] Fawcett RG. Acute psychosis associated with anti-NMDA-receptor antibodies and bilateral ovarian teratomas: a case report. J Clin Psychiatry. 2010;**71**(4):504. doi:10.4088/JCP.09l05609yel

[145] Benros ME, Mortensen PB, Eaton WW. Autoimmune diseases and infections as risk factors for schizophrenia. Ann N Y Acad Sci. 2012;**1262**:56–66. doi:10.1111/j.1749-6632.2012.06638.x

[146] DeGiorgio LA, Konstantinov KN, Lee SC, Hardin JA, Volpe BT, Diamond B. A subset of lupus anti-DNA antibodies cross-reacts with the NR2 glutamate receptor in systemic lupus erythematosus. Nat Med. 2001;**7**(11):1189–1193.

[147] Pearlman DM, Najjar S. Meta-analysis of the association between *N*-methyl-D-aspartate receptor antibodies and schizophrenia, schizoaffective disorder, bipolar disorder, and major depressive disorder. Schizophr Res. 2014;**157**(1–3):249–258. doi:10.1016/j.schres.2014.05.001

[148] Smyth AM, Lawrie SM. The neuroimmunology of schizophrenia. Clin Psychopharmacol Neurosci. 2013;**11**(3):107–117. doi:10.9758/cpn.2013.11.3.107

[149] Deakin J, Lennox BR, Zandi MS. Antibodies to the *N*-methyl-D-aspartate receptor and other synaptic proteins in psychosis. Biol Psychiatry. 2014;**75**(4):284–291. doi:10.1016/j.biopsych.2013.07.018

[150] Steiner J, Walter M, Glanz W, Sarnyai Z, Bernstein HG, Vielhaber S, Kästner A, Skalej M, Jordan W, Schiltz K, Klingbeil C, Wandinger KP, Bogerts B, Stoecker W. Increased prevalence of diverse *N*-methyl-D-aspartate glutamate receptor antibodies in patients with an initial diagnosis of schizophrenia: specific relevance of IgG NR1a antibodies for distinction from *N*-methyl-D-aspartate glutamate receptor encephalitis. JAMA Psychiatry. 2013;**70**(3):271–278. doi:10.1001/2013.jamapsychiatry.86

[151] Zandi MS, Irani SR, Lang B, Waters P, Jones PB, McKenna P, Coles AJ, Vincent A, Lennox BR. Disease-relevant autoantibodies in first episode schizophrenia. J Neurol. 2011;**258**(4):686–688. doi:10.1007/s00415-010-5788-9

[152] Masdeu JC, González-Pinto A, Matute C, Ruiz De Azúa S, Palomino A, De Leon J, Berman KF, Dalmau J. Serum IgG antibodies against the NR1 subunit of the NMDA receptor not detected in schizophrenia. Am J Psychiatry. 2012;**169**(10):1120–1121. doi:10.1176/appi.ajp.2012.12050646

[153] Rhoads J, Guirgis H, McKnight C, Duchemin AM. Lack of anti-NMDA receptor autoantibodies in the serum of subjects with schizophrenia. Schizophr Res. 2011;**129**(2–3):213–214. doi:10.1016/j.schres.2010.12.018

[154] Tsutsui K, Kanbayashi T, Tanaka K, Boku S, Ito W, Tokunaga J, Mori A, Hishikawa Y, Shimizu T, Nishino S. Anti-NMDA-receptor antibody detected in encephalitis, schizophrenia, and narcolepsy with psychotic features. BMC Psychiatry. 2012;**12**:37. doi:10.1186/1471-244X-12-37

[155] Coyle JT. NMDA receptor and schizophrenia: a brief history. Schizophr Bull. 2012;**38**(5):920–926. doi:10.1093/schbul/sbs076

[156] Belforte JE, Zsiros V, Sklar ER, Jiang Z, Yu G, Li Y, Quinlan EM, Nakazawa K. Postnatal NMDA receptor ablation in corticolimbic interneurons confers schizophrenia-like phenotypes. Nat Neurosci. 2010;**13**(1):76–83. doi:10.1038/nn.2447

[157] Timms AE, Dorschner MO, Wechsler J, Choi KY, Kirkwood R, Girirajan S, Baker C, Eichler EE, Korvatska O, Roche KW, Horwitz MS, Tsuang DW. Support for the *N*-methyl-D-aspartate receptor hypofunction hypothesis of schizophrenia from exome sequencing in multiplex families. JAMA Psychiatry. 2013;**70**(6):582–590. doi:10.1001/jamapsychiatry.2013.1195

[158] Pilowsky LS, Bressan RA, Stone JM, Erlandsson K, Mulligan RS, Krystal JH, Ell PJ. First *in vivo* evidence of an NMDA receptor deficit in medication-free schizophrenic patients. Mol Psychiatry. 2006;**11**(2):118–119. doi:10.1038/sj.mp.4001751

[159] Pomarol-Clotet E, Honey GD, Murray GK, Corlett PR, Absalom AR, Lee M, McKenna PJ, Bullmore ET, Fletcher PC. Psychological effects of ketamine in healthy volunteers. Phenomenological study. Br J Psychiatry. 2006;**189**:173–179. doi:10.1192/bjp.bp.105.015263

[160] Javitt DC. Glutamate and schizophrenia: phencyclidine, *N*-methyl-D-aspartate receptors, and dopamine-glutamate interactions. Int Rev Neurobiol. 2007;**78**:69–108.

[161] Fromer M, Pocklington AJ, Kavanagh DH, Williams HJ, Dwyer S, Gormley P, Georgieva L, Rees E, Palta P, Ruderfer DM, Carrera N, Humphreys I, Johnson JS, Roussos P, Barker DD, Banks E, Milanova V, Grant SG, Hannon E, Rose SA, Chambert K, Mahajan M, Scolnick EM, Moran JL, Kirov G, Palotie A, McCarroll SA, Holmans P, Sklar P, Owen MJ, Purcell SM, O'Donovan MC. *De novo* mutations in schizophrenia implicate synaptic networks. Nature. 2014;**506**(7487):179–184. doi:10.1038/nature12929

[162] Prüss H, Finke C, Höltje M, Hofmann J, Klingbeil C, Probst C, Borowski K, Ahnert-Hilger G, Harms L, Schwab JM, Ploner CJ, Komorowski L, Stoecker W, Dalmau J, Wandinger KP. *N*-methyl-D-aspartate receptor antibodies in herpes simplex encephalitis. Ann Neurol. 2012;**72**(6):902–911. doi:10.1002/ana.23689

[163] Hammer C, Stepniak B, Schneider A, Papiol S, Tantra M, Begemann M, Sirén AL, Pardo LA, Sperling S, Mohd Jofrry S, Gurvich A, Jensen N, Ostmeier K, Lühder F, Probst C, Martens H, Gillis M, Saher G, Assogna F, Spalletta G, Stöcker W, Schulz TF, Nave KA, Ehrenreich H. Neuropsychiatric disease relevance of circulating anti-NMDA receptor autoantibodies depends on blood-brain barrier integrity. Mol Psychiatry. 2014;**19**(10):1143–1149. doi:10.1038/mp.2013.110

[164] Kannan G, Crawford JA, Yang C, Gressitt KL, Ihenatu C, Krasnova IN, Cadet JL, Yolken RH, Severance EG, Pletnikov MV. Anti-NMDA receptor autoantibodies and associated neurobehavioral pathology in mice are dependent on age of first exposure to *Toxoplasma gondii*. Neurobiol Dis. 2016;**91**:307–314. doi:10.1016/j.nbd.2016.03.005

[165] Freedman R. Schizophrenia. N Engl J Med. 2003;**349**(18):1738–1749.

[166] Cardno AG, Marshall EJ, Coid B, Macdonald AM, Ribchester TR, Davies NJ, Venturi P, Jones LA, Lewis SW, Sham PC, Gottesman II, Farmer AE, McGuffin P, Reveley AM, Murray RM. Heritability estimates for psychotic disorders: the Maudsley twin psychosis series. Arch Gen Psychiatry. 1999;**56**(2):162–168. doi:10.1001/archpsyc.56.2.162

[167] Fatemi SH, Pearce DA, Brooks AI, Sidwell RW. Prenatal viral infection in mouse causes differential expression of genes in brains of mouse progeny: a potential animal model for schizophrenia and autism. Synapse. 2005;**57**(2):91–99. doi:10.1002/syn.20162

[168] Harrison PJ, Owen MJ. Genes for schizophrenia? Recent findings and their pathophysiological implications. Lancet. 2003;**361**(9355):417–419. doi:10.1016/S0140-6736(03)12379-3

[169] Carter CJ. Schizophrenia: a pathogenetic autoimmune disease caused by viruses and pathogens and dependent on genes. J Pathog. 2011;**2011**:128318. doi:10.4061/2011/128318

[170] Tomonaga K. Virus-induced neurobehavioral disorders: mechanisms and implications. Trends Mol Med. 2004;**10**(2):71–77. doi:10.1016/j.molmed.2003.12.001

[171] Harrison PJ, Law AJ. Neuregulin 1 and schizophrenia: Genetics, gene expression, and neurobiology. Biol Psychiatry. 2006;**60**(2):132–140. doi:10.1016/j.biopsych.2005.11.002

[172] Rico B, Marín O. Neuregulin signaling, cortical circuitry development and schizophrenia. Curr Opin Genet Dev. 201;**21**(3):262–270. doi:10.1016/j.gde.2010.12.010

[173] Chen CY, Lu RB, Yeh YW, Shih MC, Huang SY. Association study of catechol-O-methyltransferase gene polymorphisms with schizophrenia and psychopathological symptoms in Han Chinese. Genes Brain Behav. 2011;**10**(3):316–324. doi:10.1111/j. 1601-183X.2010.00670.x

[174] Willis A, Bender HU, Steel G, Valle D. PRODH variants and risk for schizophrenia. Amino Acids. 2008;**35**(4):673–679. doi:10.1007/s00726-008-0111-0

[175] Voisey J, Swagell CD, Hughes IP, Connor JP, Lawford BR, Young RM, Morris CP. A polymorphism in the dysbindin gene (DTNBP1) associated with multiple psychiatric disorders including schizophrenia. Behav Brain Funct. 2010;**6**(1):41. doi:10.1186/1744-9081-6-41

[176] Ding L, Hegde AN. Expression of RGS4 splice variants in dorsolateral prefrontal cortex of schizophrenic and bipolar disorder patients. Biol Psychiatry. 2009;**65**(6):541–545. doi:10.1016/j.biopsych.2008.10.026

[177] Ritsner M, Modai I, Ziv H, Amir S, Halperin T, Weizman A, Navon R. An association of CAG repeats at the KCNN3 locus with symptom dimensions of schizophrenia. Biol Psychiatry. 2002;**51**(10):788–794. doi:10.1016/S0006-3223(01)01348-8

[178] Madeira C, Freitas ME, Vargas-Lopes C, Wolosker H, Panizzutti R. Increased brain D-amino acid oxidase (DAAO) activity in schizophrenia. Schizophr Res. 2008; **101**(1–3):76–83. doi:10.1016/j.schres.2008.02.002

[179] Carter CJ. Schizophrenia susceptibility genes directly implicated in the life cycles of pathogens: cytomegalovirus, influenza, herpes simplex, rubella, and *Toxoplasma gondii*. Schizophr Bull. 2009;**35**(6):1163–1182. doi:10.1093/schbul/sbn054

[180] Carter CJ. Toxoplasmosis and polygenic disease susceptibility genes: extensive *Toxoplasma gondii* host/pathogen interactome enrichment in nine psychiatric or neurological disorders. J Pathog. 2013;**2013**:965046. doi:10.1155/2013/965046

[181] Pearce BD. Schizophrenia and viral infection during neurodevelopment: a focus on mechanisms. Mol Psychiatry. 2001;**6**(6):634–646. doi:10.1038/sj.mp.4000956

[182] Tsuang MT, Stone WS, Faraone SV. Genes, environment and schizophrenia. Br J Psychiatry Suppl. 2001;**178**(40):s18–s24. doi:10.1192/bjp.178.40.s18

[183] Khan IA, Murphy PM, Casciotti L, Schwartzman JD, Collins J, Gao JL, Yeaman GR. Mice lacking the chemokine receptor CCR1 show increased susceptibility to *Toxoplasma gondii* infection. J Immunol. 2001;**166**(3):1930–1937. doi:10.4049/jimmunol.166.3.1930

[184] Yap GS, Ortmann R, Shevach E, Sher A. A heritable defect in IL-12 signaling in B10.Q/J mice. II. Effect on acute resistance to *Toxoplasma gondii* and rescue by IL-18 treatment. J Immunol. 2001;**166**(9):5720–5725. doi:10.4049/jimmunol.166.9.5720

[185] Mack DG, Johnson JJ, Roberts F, Roberts CW, Estes RG, David C, Grumet FC, McLeod R. HLA-class II genes modify outcome of *Toxoplasma gondii* infection. Int J Parasitol. 1999;**29**(9):1351–1358. doi:10.1016/S0020-7519(99)00152-6

[186] Suzuki Y, Wong SY, Grumet FC, Fessel J, Montoya JG, Zolopa AR, Portmore A, Schumacher-Perdreau F, Schrappe M, Köppen S, Ruf B, Brown BW, Remington JS. Evidence for genetic regulation of susceptibility to toxoplasmic encephalitis in AIDS patients. J Infect Dis. 1996;**173**(1):265–268. doi:10.1093/infdis/173.1.265

[187] Avramopoulos D, Pearce BD, McGrath J, Wolyniec P, Wang R, Eckart N, Hatzimanolis A, Goes FS, Nestadt G, Mulle J, Coneely K, Hopkins M, Ruczinski I, Yolken R, Pulver AE. Infection and inflammation in schizophrenia and bipolar disorder: a genome wide study for interactions with genetic variation. PLoS One. 2015;**10**(3):e0116696. doi:10.1371/journal.pone.0116696

[188] Børglum AD, Demontis D, Grove J, Pallesen J, Hollegaard MV, Pedersen CB, Hedemand A, Mattheisen M, Uitterlinden A, Nyegaard M, Ørntoft T, Wiuf C, Didriksen M, Nordentoft M, Nöthen MM, Rietschel M, Ophoff RA, Cichon S, Yolken RH, Hougaard DM, Mortensen PB, Mors O. Genome-wide study of association and interaction with maternal cytomegalovirus infection suggests new schizophrenia loci. Mol Psychiatry. 2014;**19**(3):325–333. doi:10.1038/mp.2013.2

[189] Kannan G, Sawa A, Pletnikov MV. Mouse models of gene-environment interactions in schizophrenia. Neurobiol Dis. 2013;**57**:5–11. doi:10.1016/j.nbd.2013.05.012

[190] Kim T, Kim HJ, Park JK, Kim JW, Chung JH. Association between polymorphisms of arachidonate 12-lipoxygenase (ALOX12) and schizophrenia in a Korean population. Behav Brain Funct. 2010;**6**:44. doi:10.1186/1744-9081-6-44

[191] Witola WH, Liu SR, Montpetit A, Welti R, Hypolite M, Roth M, Zhou Y, Mui E, Cesbron-Delauw MF, Fournie GJ, Cavailles P, Bisanz C, Boyer K, Withers S, Noble AG, Swisher CN, Heydemann PT, Rabiah P, Muench SP, McLeod R. ALOX12 in human toxoplasmosis. Infect Immun. 2014;**82**(7):2670–2679. doi:10.1128/IAI.01505-13

[192] Lang F, Strutz-Seebohm N, Seebohm G, Lang UE. Significance of SGK1 in the regulation of neuronal function. J Physiol. 2010;**588**(Pt 18):3349–3354. doi:10.1113/jphysiol.2010.190926

[193] Anacker C, Cattaneo A, Musaelyan K, Zunszain PA, Horowitz M, Molteni R, Luoni A, Calabrese F, Tansey K, Gennarelli M, Thuret S, Price J, Uher R, Riva MA, Pariante CM. Role for the kinase SGK1 in stress, depression, and glucocorticoid effects on hippocampal neurogenesis. Proc Natl Acad Sci U S A. 2013;**110**(21):8708–8713. doi:10.1073/pnas.1300886110

[194] Kadkhodaei B, Ito T, Joodmardi E, Mattsson B, Rouillard C, Carta M, Muramatsu S, Sumi-Ichinose C, Nomura T, Metzger D, Chambon P, Lindqvist E, Larsson NG, Olson L, Björklund A, Ichinose H, Perlmann T. Nurr1 is required for maintenance of matur-

ing and adult midbrain dopamine neurons. J Neurosci. 2009;**29**(50):15923–15932. doi:10.1523/JNEUROSCI.3910-09.2009

[195] Eells JB, Varela-Stokes A, Guo-Ross SX, Kummari E, Smith HM, Cox E, Lindsay DS. Chronic *Toxoplasma gondii* in Nurr1-null heterozygous mice exacerbates elevated open field activity. PLoS One. 2015;**10**(4):e0119280. doi:10.1371/journal.pone.0119280

[196] Mullonkal CJ, Toledo-Pereyra LH. Akt in ischemia and reperfusion. J Invest Surg. 2007;**20**(3):195–203. doi:10.1080/08941930701366471

[197] Tan HY, Nicodemus KK, Chen Q, Li Z, Brooke JK, Honea R, Kolachana BS, Straub RE, Meyer-Lindenberg A, Sei Y, Mattay VS, Callicott JH, Weinberger DR. Genetic variation in AKT1 is linked to dopamine-associated prefrontal cortical structure and function in humans. J Clin Invest. 2008;**118**(6):2200–2208. doi:10.1172/JCI34725

[198] Fellerhoff B, Laumbacher B, Mueller N, Gu S, Wank R. Associations between *Chlamydophila* infections, schizophrenia and risk of HLA-A10. Mol Psychiatry. 2007;**12**(3):264–272. doi:10.1038/sj.mp.4001925

[199] Kim JJ, Shirts BH, Dayal M, Bacanu SA, Wood J, Xie W, Zhang X, Chowdari KV, Yolken R, Devlin B, Nimgaonkar VL. Are exposure to cytomegalovirus and genetic variation on chromosome 6p joint risk factors for schizophrenia? Ann Med. 2007;**39**(2):145–153. doi:10.1080/07853890601083808

[200] Prasad KM, Bamne MN, Shirts BH, Goradia D, Mannali V, Pancholi KM, Xue B, McClain L, Yolken RH, Keshavan MS, Nimgaonkar VL. Grey matter changes associated with host genetic variation and exposure to herpes simplex virus 1 (HSV1) in first episode schizophrenia. Schizophr Res. 2010;**118**(1–3):232–239. doi:10.1016/j.schres.2010.01.007

[201] Shirts BH, Kim JJ, Reich S, Dickerson FB, Yolken RH, Devlin B, Nimgaonkar VL. Polymorphisms in MICB are associated with human herpes virus seropositivity and schizophrenia risk. Schizophr Res. 2007;**94**(1–3):342–353. doi:10.1016/j.schres.2007.04.021

[202] Kusbeci OY, Miman O, Yaman M, Aktepe OC, Yazar S. Could *Toxoplasma gondii* have any role in Alzheimer disease? Alzheimer Dis Assoc Disord. 2011;**25**(1):1–3. doi:10.1097/WAD.0b013e3181f73bc2

[203] Miman O, Kusbeci OY, Aktepe OC, Cetinkaya Z. The probable relation between *Toxoplasma gondii* and Parkinson's disease. Neurosci Lett. 2010;**475**(3):129–131. doi:10.1016/j.neulet.2010.03.057

[204] Yazar S, Arman F, Yalçin S, Demirtas F, Yaman O, Sahin I. Investigation of probable relationship between *Toxoplasma gondii* and cryptogenic epilepsy. Seizure. 2003;**12**(2):107–109. doi:10.1016/S1059-1311(02)00256-X

[205] Webster JP, Kaushik M, Bristow GC, McConkey GA. *Toxoplasma gondii* infection, from predation to schizophrenia: can animal behaviour help us understand human behaviour? J Exp Biol. 2013;**216**(Pt 1):99–112. doi:10.1242/jeb.074716.

[206] Fond G, Boyer L, Gaman A, Laouamri H, Attiba D, Richard JR, Delavest M, Houenou J, Le Corvoisier P, Charron D, Krishnamoorthy R, Oliveira J, Tamouza R, Yolken R, Dickerson F, Leboyer M, Hamdani N. Treatment with anti-toxoplasmic activity (TATA) for toxoplasma positive patients with bipolar disorders or schizophrenia: a cross-sectional study. J Psychiatr Res. 2015;**63**:58–64. doi:10.1016/j.jpsychires.2015.02.011

Chapter 5

Cognitive Biases in Schizophrenia Spectrum Disorders

V. Juárez Ramos and M. L. Montánchez Torres

Additional information is available at the end of the chapter

http://dx.doi.org/10.5772/65726

Abstract

In the scientific literature, a close relationship between cognitive biases and schizophrenia disorder has been widely demonstrated. Cognitive biases would be a pattern of deviation in judgment, in which the inferences we make about other people and/or situations can be illogical. Throughout this chapter will be analyzed how some cognitive biases are greatly related and are involved in the onset, maintenance, relapse and recovery of this disorder. Specifically, we will discuss five biases [need for closure, overconfidence bias, bias against confirmatory evidence (BACE), bias against disconfirmatory evidence (BADE) and above all jumping to conclusions (JTC)] that have been extensively studied and shown in patients with schizophrenia, especially with delusions. In this chapter the importance of studying in depth these cognitive biases in schizophrenia in order to understand, reduce and avoid them will be seen. The reduction and avoidance of these biases will result in an improvement in symptoms of schizophrenia. Therefore, it will lead to a faster, effective recovery. Moreover, the patient with schizophrenia will have an active role in his recovery. As a result, nowadays we can find several behavioral cognitive therapies, which are working on the reduction and avoidance of these cognitive biases and are demonstrating their effectiveness.

Keywords: cognitive bias, schizophrenia, jumping to conclusions, overconfidence bias, need for closure

1. Introduction

Throughout this chapter we will focus on the great influence of some cognitive biases in the study of schizophrenia disorder. In this chapter we will describe how these cognitive biases are involved in the cognitive processes, which lead to the onset, maintenance and recover of this disorder. Therefore, we will mark the importance of studying these biases to understand, reduce and avoid them. As a result, this knowledge would produce an improvement of the symptoms of schizophrenia, increasing the quality of life of these patients.

Schizophrenia is a mental disorder characterized by a set of psychotic disorders which usually involve abnormal social behavior and cognitive deficit [1]. Schizophrenia includes environmental and genetic factors. In general, the onset of this disorder would be due to environmental factors such as stress, cannabis, poor nutrition during pregnant and some traumatic episodes or infections, among others [2]. Genetic factors include a variety of common and rare genetic variants [3]. However, the genetic influence must be studied in the context of interaction with environmental, social and cognitive effects [4].

In general, the symptoms of schizophrenia are usually divided into two main groups: positive or negative psychotic symptoms. However, these disorders also have other important aspects, which must be observed such as behavioral, affective and cognitive symptoms [5].

On the one hand, the positive symptoms would be typified by failure to understand what is real. In this category we will find, for example, delusions, hallucinations and disorganized speech. On the other hand, the negative symptoms would be typified by diminished emotional expression or avolition such as apathy or alogia. The emotional symptoms would be affective flattening, dysphoria and depression, among others. The behavioral symptoms would be hostility, impulsivity, aggressive attitudes and antisocial behavior [6, 7]. And finally, cognitive symptoms would include cognitive deficits, for example, in the executive functions [1]. In 2013, the American Psychiatric Association removed all subclassifications of schizophrenia in the new publication of DSM-5 [8].

Focusing in the factors which are involved in the onset and maintenance of schizophrenia disorder, many studies have found multiple implicated psychological mechanisms. However, we will talk about some implied cognitive biases such as jumping to conclusions (JTC) and overconfidence bias, among others.

In 1974, Tervsky and Kahneman defined the term of cognitive bias [9]. In a general definition, we can say that a cognitive bias would be a pattern of deviation in judgment, in which the inferences we make about other people and/or situations can be illogical [10]. Besides, diverse studies have found that these cognitive biases can be influenced by the context, personal motivation, failure in the information processing and social/culture factors [11, 12].

In schizophrenia research, throughout years cognitive behavioral models have established a strong relationship between some cognitive biases and schizophrenia disorders especially in those patients with positive symptomatology [13, 14]. One of the origins and maintenance of delusions are the cognitive biases or deficits in probabilistic reasoning processes of individuals.

However, these biases have been also studied in healthy populations with high scores on schizotypy [13]. Schizotypy would be qualitatively analogous but quantitatively more moderate than schizophrenia. Schizotypy trait could give us a possible explanation about the possible etiological mechanisms underlying schizophrenia spectrum disorders and may permit us to get better strategies for prevention and early detection of this disorder. Diverse studies have found that people with high schizotypy trait have more probability to display these cognitive biases [13].

In addition, several cognitive biases have been identified in those with the diagnosis or those at risk, especially when under stress or in confusing situations [15]. Therefore, it is necessary to know how these cognitive biases work in the onset, maintenance and relapse or recovery from this disorder.

Following this line, multiple studies have found bidirectional effects in these cognitive biases, that is, one bias or its results could influence another bias or the effects of that second bias and vice versa [16]. For example, Buchy et al. [17] investigated the relationship between jumping to conclusions (JTC) bias and bias against disconfirmatory evidence (BADE) based on the dimensional model of schizophrenia which bodes unifying cognitive biases or that these cognitive biases may combine to contribute to the formation of the delusional aspects of psychosis. Having said that, it is easy supposing there will have combinations of cognitive biases that together would be involved in the onset, maintenance, relapse and/or recovery from this disorder.

Another enriching way of studying cognitive biases in schizophrenia is through the comparison between the involved cognitive biases in other mental disorders. This study may give us important clues. For example, we could know how these operate in different mental disorders and its symptoms. In fact, we could find specific cognitive biases, which are implicated in a mental disorder but not in other disorders. An example of this type of studio, which tried to compare some psychiatric disorders and its relationship with the cognitive biases, was carried out by Wittorf et al. [18]. These authors did a cross-sectional study about jumping to conclusion (JTC) and attributional biases (AB) with 20 patients with paranoid schizophrenia, 20 patients with depression, 15 patients with anorexia nervosa and 55 nonclinical controls. Participants completed a modified version of the beads task, a revised German version of the Internal, Personal and Situational Attributions Questionnaire (AB) and several symptoms and neurocognitive measures. The findings showed that patients with schizophrenia evidenced that they are more likely to exhibit a jumping to conclusions bias than the other groups (patients with depression or anorexia nervosa and healthy controls). With respect to attentional bias, there were no significant differences between the clinical groups in personalizing bias, but patients with schizophrenia exhibited greater externalizing than the other clinical groups. The innovation of this studio is that it compared two cognitive biases in different psychiatric disorders and this can help us in understanding them better. Therefore, the ultimate purpose of the study of cognitive biases and their influence on schizophrenia is to better understand how these biases are involved in cognitive processes of patients with schizophrenia and how we can get to avoid, know and reduce them. This will result in a recovery of this disorder more effective and faster. In addition, we will achieve an active role of the patient with schizophrenia in his recovery and prevention of a possible relapse. Due to this multiple cognitive behavioral therapies work on the avoidance and reduction of cognitive biases in their programs. For instance, we can name the metacognitive training/therapy [19] or the famous cognitive bias modification therapy [20]. The objective of these therapies is to detect, reduce and avoid the cognitive bias implicated in the onset and maintenance of schizophrenia in order to get an effective recovery and preventing a relapse. For that, different modules are used to work in different biases where the patient knows the bias, becomes aware of it and works on its reduction and avoidance.

2. Schizophrenia and cognitive biases

As mentioned above, some cognitive biases have been widely related to schizophrenia such as need for closure [21], overconfidence bias [14], bias against confirmatory evidence (BACE), bias against disconfirmatory evidence (BADE) and above all jumping to conclusions [13, 17]. Then we will explain these four cognitive biases and their relationship with this disorder.

2.1. Jumping to conclusions, against disconfirmatory evidence bias (BADE) and bias against confirmatory evidence (BACE)

The jumping to conclusions is a cognitive bias where there is a data-gathering bias and a contrast of hypothesis testing bias. This cognitive bias occurs when there is a tendency to make decisions very quickly even when there may not be a lot of evidence [22]. This bias is usually tested using probabilistic reasoning tasks based on a Bayesian model of probabilistic inference [13, 23]. As it is stated above, jumping to conclusions bias is a bias which has been largely related to patients with schizophrenia, especially, in patients with delusions [13, 17].

Numerous researches said that jumping to conclusions would be an endophenotype of psychosis [24]. In support of this, Menon et al. [25] found that antipsychotic treatment in patients with schizophrenia did not reduce the bias which may suggest that jumping to conclusions bias could be a trait maker for schizophrenia. This bias has also been observed in first-degree relatives of patients with schizophrenia above all patients with delusions [26]. Similarly, these cognitive biases have been observed in patients with psychosis.

The jumping to conclusions bias is closely related to the origin and maintenance of delusions. In fact, most studies have found this bias in patients with schizophrenia who have positive symptoms and not in patients with schizophrenia who have a negative symptomatology. Therefore, this bias is more associated with the delusions rather than with schizophrenia disorder [26]. The JTC is found in people with delusions with a schizophrenia diagnosis or delusional disorder. The subjects with delusions show a bias in the collection of information. They need fewer data than the normal population to reach to a final decision. In delirium process, there is a development constant by which ideas confirm and disconfirm through approaches to hypothesis, information gathering and contrast of the results with the previous hypothesis. Probably some of these steps are inadequate in delusional patients, both cognitive and emotional processes.

At present, two different hypotheses have been advanced to explain this cognitive bias [27]. On the one hand, several authors support the hypothesis that people with jumping to conclusions bias overestimate the conviction in their choices at the beginning of the decision process [28]. In line with this viewpoint, patients with schizophrenia tend to accept choices early that wrong inferences may.

On the other hand, other authors argue that the bias could be due to a low information threshold for acceptance of a decision [29]. "The hypothesis of liberal acceptance" was proposed by Moritz and Woodward [30]. These authors based on their hypothesis in the decrement of confidence gap in patients with schizophrenia who made final decisions with little evidence collected for them. Moreover, liberal acceptance is thought as core deficit because it is exhibited in delusion-relevant scenarios and neutral settings. Different experimental tasks have been used to support their hypothesis. For example, Moritz et al. [31] carried out an experiment called "Who wants to be a millionaire?," a TV game, in patients with schizophrenia and healthy control where they were asked to rate the probability of each of four response alternatives to general knowledge questions. The results showed that patients reached to final decisions at 54 % subjective probability ratings and healthy controls at 70 %.

In addition, several studies have explored the possible relationship between jumping to conclusion bias and the bias against disconfirmatory evidence (BADE) and bias against confirmatory evidence (BACE) [13, 17].

Bias against disconfirmatory evidence (BADE) is a cognitive bias where, regardless of the inconsistent information, the hypothesis holds despite evidence to the contrary. Conversely, in the bias against confirmatory evidence (BACE) individuals, regardless of inconsistent information, they maintain their belief or hypothesis because of the evidence in favor of it [32]. The dimensional model of schizophrenia predicts unifying cognitive biases or combined cognitive biases to contribute toward the formation of the delusional aspects of psychosis [17]. For example, according to Munz [33], jumping to conclusions would play a facilitating role in the formation of new delusional systems and BADE. This dimensional model emphasizes quantitative gradations of psychopathology, both within and between subjects, rather than qualitative, discrete, all-or-none class distinctions. However, nowadays the relationship between these remains unclear because the studies are controversial and there is no consensus. At present, it is unclear whether these reasoning biases share common underpinnings or are independent [33].

Based on the previous results of several studies about schizophrenia research [17, 32, 34], our team decided to study the jumping to conclusion bias, bias against disconfirmatory evidence (BADE) and bias against confirmatory evidence (BACE) in patients with schizophrenia and healthy population with high and low score in schizotypy [13] using the Pictures Decision Task [13, 23]. Following the dimensional theory of schizophrenia, we thought that it was interesting to study the population with high schizotypy since it would be useful to understand the etiological mechanisms that there are under schizophrenia spectrum disorders. This understanding could do progress to the own prevention or the early detection of these disorders [35]. The schizotypy is found within the normal variation of population general. Individuals with high schizotypy have a similar psychopathology and cognitive styles than patients with schizophrenia, that is, they are similar qualitatively but they are not similar quantitatively to patients with schizophrenia [13]. For that, we recruited a total of 45 participants divided in three groups: 15 patients with schizophrenia and 30 healthy participants (15 high schizotypy and 15 low schizotypy). To measure schizotypy, we used the Community Assessment of Psychic Experiences (CAPE) [36]. Moreover, there are no significant differences between them in age, education, gender, or premorbid intelligence. Once participants were tested, they performed the Pictures Decision Task.

The results of the experiment demonstrated that the patients with schizophrenia displayed jumping to conclusions more easily than control groups (high and low schizotypy). Also, patients with schizophrenia showed confirmatory bias, so that, they were more reticent to change their hypothesis even though it would have new disconfirmatory evidence. Moreover, patients with schizophrenia were less sensitive to the feedback, so they did less use of feedback. For example, in the cue condition, they did not profit in possible solutions when the other two control groups (high and low schizotypy) did it. Therefore, we suggested that jumping to conclusions bias may be related to propensity to hold strong beliefs (high plausibility rating at first stages) and/or to low feedback sensitivity (FS), above all, when the task or context is more ambiguous and difficult (uncued trials). This is corroborated by the fact that all groups reproduced jumping to conclusions in the cued condition, but not in the uncued condition (difficult task), where the patients with schizophrenia and high schizotypy group reproduced the bias more early than low schizotypy group.

Based on these results, we could conclude that jumping to conclusions bias was a general bias because this bias is not only presented in schizophrenia but also in nonclinical population (high- and low-schizotypy healthy populations). However, patients with schizophrenia would show it earlier and stronger than healthy population. It could say that jumping to conclusions bias would be found in a straight line where the patients with schizophrenia would have a greater tendency to show it, followed by populations with high schizotypy and low schizotypy. Furthermore, this line would be influenced by context (more or less ambiguity). Hence, using a controlled or heuristic processing would depend on context and type of participant. Also, we observed that feedback sensitivity could be a factor that affects this bias. However, there is no relationship between jumping to conclusions bias and the two other biases [bias against disconfirmatory evidence (BADE) and bias against confirmatory evidence (BACE)].

To conclude, these results can have an important implication since they could help in the treatment, prevention, or recovery from schizophrenia. For example, the therapy X could try to teach how does more effective hypothesis testing through making a better use of feedback. The jumping to conclusions bias and the other two biases could represent an important therapeutic target. Individual differences in JTC performance could be useful in determining the best course of treatment. Training programs that aim to ameliorate the jumping to conclusions response style might prove to be an important adjunct to established therapies [37]. An example of this, we can find it with the metacognitive training/therapy [19]. This therapy works on different aspects between the cognitive biases like jumping to conclusions or confirmatory bias. In this therapy there are sixteen modules, which must be done by the patient with schizophrenia. For example, to work the confirmation bias, module 3 is used where patients are informed and explained about this bias and then performed different tasks. A typical task to work this bias would consist in a task with a series of three pictures which are shown in reversed order. The sequences of pictures gradually reveal an ambiguous plot. For each picture, participants are asked to rate the plausibility of four different interpretations. The goal of this task is that patients learn to look for more information before making a judgment and therefore avoiding the confirmation or disconfirmation bias [17, 37].

2.2. Need for closure bias

Another cognitive bias that has been linked to schizophrenia disorder is the need for closure bias [21, 38]. However, as discussed below this bias has not been studied so deeply as the other biases (jumping to conclusions, BACE and BADE). Therefore, its influence in schizophrenia disorder is not well known yet. Moreover, there are not many studies on its bidirectional relationship with the other implicated cognitive biases in the schizophrenia.

According to Kruglanski [39], the cognitive bias called need for closure is:

> "the need to reach a fast decision to have an answer and to escape the feeling of doubt and uncertainty and "freeze" by failing to update".

In addition, this author later adds that this bias could be displayed through the desire for predictability and preference for order and structure and discomfort with ambiguity (need for closure [40]). In general, different studies have evidenced that people who show the need for closure bias have a great need for cognitive closure. They dislike uncertainty and prefer to reach conclusions quickly and with certainty [39–42].

According to Federico et al. [41]:

> "They seek to accomplish this goal by "seizing" quickly on any available information to reach conclusions and by "freezing" on these conclusions once they are reached".

Focusing in the study of this bias in schizophrenia, Colbert and Peters [38] demonstrated that members of the general population that are delusion prone had a higher score on the need for closure scale (NCS). Moreover, these individuals displayed jumping to conclusions bias. So they concluded that as the data-gathering reasoning bias was found in delusion-prone individuals, this suggests that it may be involved in the formation, rather than merely the maintenance, of delusional beliefs.

In other study, McKay et al. [21] found this bias in patients with schizophrenia. On the other hand, the results of this investigation showed that need for closure and jumping to conclusions biases would not seem related with each other. The intolerance of ambiguity correlated positively with delusion proneness and decisiveness correlated negatively. According to these authors, the delusion-prone individuals would be more indecisive in everyday life. In addition, the need for closure has been associated with jumping to conclusions since the intolerance to ambiguity contexts would lead to jumping to conclusions [21]. The following year, in 2007, these authors realized other experiments studying the relationship between need for closure and schizophrenia [43]. They wanted to replicate the study of Bentall and Swarbrick [44].

Bentall and Swarbrick thought that patients with delusions may be highly intolerant of ambiguity, that is, they show need for closure and in point the fact that the results of their study confirmed their hypothesis. They found that patients with delusions were highly intolerant of ambiguity and had a higher score in the need for closure scale (NCS). Based on this studio, McKay et al. [43] hypothesized that 22 patients with a history of persecutory delusions would exhibit higher need for closure and a more extreme jumping to conclusions bias than 19 healthy control participants. For that, the participants must realize a probabilistic task and fill out depression and need for closure scale. The results demonstrated that patients with persecutory delusions had a higher score than healthy control group. Therefore, the results support an association between persecutory delusions and need for closure. In addition, they did not find relationship between jumping to conclusions and need for closure.

Within the relationships between cognitive biases (e.g., jumping to conclusions, bias against disconfirmatory evidence, need for closure), we can find the interesting study of Moritz et al. [45]. These authors studied a total of 56 patients with schizophrenia through four independent components: jumping to conclusions, personalizing attributional style, inflexibility and low self-esteem. The study lends tentative support for the claim that candidate cognitive mechanisms for delusions only partially overlap, so these mechanisms must be more widely studied in order to have a higher knowledge. Meantime, these authors propose that these biases should be treated independently via behavioral cognitive therapies, which work these biases.

Analyzing all these studies, we see clearly that it is necessary to study more deeply the need for closure and its implication in schizophrenia. Nowadays, it is not known how this bias works in schizophrenia, that is, it is not clear what is its real involvement in the onset, maintenance and relapse of schizophrenia disorder. In fact, if we try to find studies, we will encounter that there are few or almost no one study which attempts to discern what is its influence on schizophrenia. In addition, there are few studies that have tried to investigate the relationship of the implicated cognitive biases in schizophrenia. If the relationship between them is independent, dependent or partially dependent is unclear. In general, it seems that these biases are independent but it is necessary to study better. What is clear is that these cognitive biases play an important role in schizophrenia because they have been found in the same population. In conclusion, the study of need for closure bias and its influence on schizophrenia is needed. In addition, the relationship between these biases in order to obtain better effective therapies should be also examined. While this is not achieved as it is said by Moritz et al. [45], these cognitive biases should be treated independently in the therapies.

2.3. Overconfidence bias

Finally, another cognitive bias that has been related to schizophrenia disorder is overconfidence bias [46] because the patients with schizophrenia displayed overconfidence in their choices or interpretations [13, 46, 47]. The overconfidence bias is the tendency to overestimate or exaggerate our own ability [48]. The response confidence is usually enhanced for erroneous judgments in patients with schizophrenia in comparison with healthy controls [13, 14]. In general, the overconfidence bias has been obtained across memory tasks [46, 47]. For example, Peters et al. [49] did an investigation with 27 patients with schizophrenia and 24 healthy controls where they were administrated a developed emotional video paradigm with 5 videos differing in emotionality (positive, 2 negative, neutral and delusional related). After each video, the participants had to do a recognition task. Also, they are asked to say the confidence

http://dx.doi.org/10.5772/65726

response, that is, participants must make old-new discriminations along with confidence ratings. The objective was to see the memory accuracy and meta-memory deficits. The results demonstrated that in the positive video the patients recognized fewer correct items than healthy controls. The patients with schizophrenia exhibited more high-confident responses for misses and false memories. So the overconfidence bias displayed by them would be related to higher probability of committing error judgments.

Also, this cognitive bias has been observed in social cognition tasks [50]. Köther et al. [50] carried out a study with 76 patients with schizophrenia or schizoaffective disorder and 30 healthy control participants. In this study, the participants must fill out the Reading the Mind in the Eyes test (Eyes test). Moreover, they had to complement a rating scale requesting response confidence. The results showed that patients with schizophrenia had more high-confidence error and fewer high-confidence correct responses. Besides, this was most clear in patients with formal thought disorder. Therefore, this study supports the implication of this cognitive bias in schizophrenia and its spectrum disorders.

Other interesting study was realized by Moritz et al. [14]. In this study, the authors analyzed the perceptual judgments in patients with schizophrenia. For that, a total of 55 patients with schizophrenia, 58 patients with obsessive-compulsive and 45 healthy controls participated. These participants had to judge whether the pictures depicted an object or not and how confident they were in this judgment. The results showed that patients with schizophrenia had more overconfidence in their error response and enhanced knowledge corruption index in comparison with healthy controls. However, accuracy score did not differ between patients with schizophrenia and obsessive-compulsive.

In the study discussed in the previous section [13] also, it was found that patients with schizophrenia showed greater confidence in the early stages of the Pictures to Decision task. In addition, they obtained more errors than healthy controls but the difference was not statistically significant. However, the overconfidence bias is a possible explanation of higher production of errors in patients with schizophrenia.

With respect to the relationship between this bias and the other implicated cognitive biases in schizophrenia, there is not a strong conclusion. In fact, as we saw in the previous cases, it is not clear if the relationship is dependent, independent, or partially dependent. Therefore, its study is necessary for higher understanding, if it is clear that this bias would be involved in the maintenance of schizophrenia disorders. Taking together the exposed results, we could intuit the important implications of these cognitive biases in the onset, maintenance and relapse or recovery in schizophrenia disorders. For that, several new therapies have been created to work in avoiding and recognizing them.

3. Conclusions

Cognitive biases have been extensively studied in patients with schizophrenia especially those with delusion-prone individuals [13, 14]. The results of experiments have shown that it is difficult to display these biases in patients with negative symptoms. So, currently the role of these cognitive biases in this disorder is not yet known exactly because they are more linked with the delusions rather than with schizophrenia disorder spectrum. The subjects with delusions show a bias in the collection of information because they need fewer data than healthy population to take a final decision.

However, it is clear that these cognitive biases have an important role in the onset, maintenance and possible relapse. Because of this important role, numerous studies have attempted to understand and see the relationship between them. But still no scientific literature agrees with the type of relationship between these cognitive biases. Although it seems that these should be interconnected through two-way relationship, studies show that the relationship between these biases is independent or as much is a partial relationship. Therefore, further study on how these biases work and how they interrelate produces greater understanding and therefore the creation of more effective therapies. Until this happens, cognitive behavioral therapies should continue to work with these cognitive biases independently. This already makes it different therapies like metacognitive training and cognitive bias modification, among others. Intervention studies of these therapies have shown satisfactory results. This type of therapy has improved recovery and avoided relapses. In addition, these therapies make the patient with schizophrenia have a more active role in their recovery, leading to greater control for patients of their disease, a better understanding of it and increased self-esteem and self-control.

In future lines must keep working on greater knowledge of cognitive biases and their relationship with each other in schizophrenia and delusional disorder. Surely, we will find new and new relationships. The ultimate goal is to get a therapy that is more effective and improve the life of these patients.

Author details

V. Juárez Ramos* and M. L. Montánchez Torres

*Address all correspondence to: juarezramosvero@hotmail.com

Education National University of Ecuador, Azogues (Cañar), Ecuador

References

[1] Hill SK, Reilly JL, Keefe RS, Gold JM, Bishop JR, Gershon ES, Tamminga CA, Pearlson GD, Keshavan MS, Sweeney JA. Mint: neuropsychological impairments in schizophrenia and psychotic bipolar disorder: findings from the Bipolar-Schizophrenia Network on Intermediate Phenotypes (B-SNIP) study. American Journal Psychiatry. 2013; 170 (11): 1275-1284. DOI: 10.1176/appi.ajp.2013.12101298

[2] Owen MJ, Sawa A, Mortensen PB. Mint: schizophrenia. Lancet. 2016; 388 (10039): 86-97. DOI: 10.1016/S0140-6736(15)01121-6

[3] Kavanagh DH, Tansey KE, O'Donovan MC, Owen MJ. Mint: schizophrenia genetics: emerging themes for a complex disorder. Molecular Psychiatry. 2014; 20 (1): 72-76. DOI: 10.1038/mp.2014.148

[4] Van Os J, Kenis G, Rutten BPF. Mint: the environment and schizophrenia. Nature. 2010; 468: 203-212. DOI: 10.1038/nature09563

[5] Van Os J, Gilvarry C, Bale R, van Horn E, Tattan T, White I, Murray R. Mint: diagnostic value of the DSM and ICD categories of psychosis: an evidence-based approach. Social Psychiatry and Psychiatric Epidemiology. 2000; 35: 305-311

[6] Hoptman MJ, Antonius D, Mauro CJ, Parker EM, Javitt DC. Mint: cortical thinning, functional connectivity and mood-related impulsivity in schizophrenia: relationship to aggressive attitudes and behavior. American Journal of Psychiatry. 2014; 171 (9): 939-948. DOI: 0.1176/appi.ajp.2014.13111553

[7] Wehring HJ, Carpenter WT. Mint: violence and schizophrenia. Schizophrenia Bulletin. 2011; 37: 877-878. DOI: 10.1093/schbul/sbr094

[8] American Psychiatric Association. Diagnostic and statistical manual of mental disorders. 5th ed. Washington: Washington, DC; 2013.

[9] Tversky A, Kahneman D. Mint: judgement under uncertainty: heuristics and biases. Science. 1974; 185: 1124-1131.

[10] Haselton MG, Nettle D andrews PW. In Buss DM editor. The Handbook of Evolutionary Psychology. Hoboken: Wiley; 2005. p. 724-746.

[11] Hilbert M. Mint: toward a synthesis of cognitive biases: how noisy information processing can bias human decision making. Psychological Bulletin. 2012; 138 (2): 211-237. DOI: 10.1037/a0025940

[12] Pfister HR, Böhm G. Mint: the multiplicity of emotions: a framework of emotional functions in decision making. Judgment and Decision Making. 2008; 3 (1): 5-17.

[13] Juárez Ramos V, Rubio JL, Delpero C, Mioni G, Stablum F, Gómez Milán E. Mint: jumping to conclusions bias, BADE and feedback sensitivity in schizophrenia and schizotypy. Consciousness and Cognition. 2014; 26: 133-144. DOI: 10.1016/j.concog.2014.03.006

[14] Moritz S, Ramdani N, Klass H andreou C, Jungclaussen D, Eifler S, Englisch S, Schirmbeck F, Zink M. Mint: overconfidence in incorrect perceptual judgments in patients with schizophrenia. Schizophrenia Research: Cognition. 2014; 1 (4): 165-170. DOI: http://dx.doi.org/10.1016/j.scog.2014.09.003

[15] Broome MR, Woolley JB, Tabraham P, Johns LC, Bramon E, Murray GK, Pariante C, McGuire PK, Murray RM. Mint: what causes the onset of psychosis?. Schizophrenia Research. 2005; 79: 23-34.

[16] Everaert J, Koster EHW, Derakshan N. Mint: the combined cognitive bias hypothesis in depression. Clinical Psychology Review. 2012; 32: 413-424. DOI: 10.1016/j.cpr.2012.04.003

[17] Buchy L, Woodward TS, Liotti M. Mint: a cognitive bias against disconfirmatory evidence (BADE) is associated with schizotypy. Schizophrenia Research. 2007; 90: 334-337. DOI: 10.1016/j.schres.2006.11.012

[18] Wittorf A., Giel KE, Hautzinger M, Rapp A, Schönenberg M, Wolkenstein L, Zipfel S, Mehl S, Fallgatter AJ, Klingberg S. Mint: specificity of jumping to conclusions and attributional biases: a comparison between patients with schizophrenia, depression and anorexia nervosa. Cognition Neuropsychiatry. 2012; 17 (3): 262-286. DOI: 10.1080/13546805.2011.633749

[19] Moritz S, Woodward TS. Mint: metacognitive training for schizophrenia patients (MCT): a pilot study on feasibility, treatment adherence and subjective efficacy. German Journal of Psychiatry. 2007a; 10: 69-78.

[20] Tran T, Hertel PT, Joormann J. Mint: cognitive bias modification: changing interpretations can alter memories. Emotion. 2001; 11 (1): 145-152.

[21] McKay R, Langdon R, Coltheart M. Mint: need for closure, jumping to conclusions and decisiveness in delusion-prone individuals. The Journal of Nervous and mental disease. 2006; 194 (6): 422-426.

[22] Huq SF, Garety PA, Hemsley DR. Mint: probabilistic judgements in deluded and non-deluded subjects. Quarterly Journal of Experimental Psychology. 1988; 40 (4): 801-812.

[23] Delpero C, Mioni G, Rubio JL, Juárez Ramos V, Gómez Milán E, Stablum F. Mint: decision making and feedback sensitivity. Journal of Cognitive Psychology. 2015; 27: 882-897. DOI: 10.1080/20445911.2015.1036759

[24] Garety P, Joyce E, Jolley S, Emsley R, Walle H, Kuipers E, Bebbington P, Fowler D, Dunn G, Freeman D. Mint: neuropsychological functioning and jumping to conclusions in delusions. Schizophrenia Research. 2013; 150 (2–3): 570-574. DOI: 10.1016/j.schres.2013.08.035

[25] Menon M, Mizrahi R, Kapur S. Mint: jumping to conclusions' and delusions in psychosis: relationship and response to treatment. Schizophrenia Research. 2008; 98: 225-231. DOI: 10.1016/j.schres.2007.08.021

[26] Van Dael F, Versmissen D, Janssen I, Myin-Germeys I, van Os J, Krabbendam L. Mint: data gathering: biased in psychosis?. Schizophrenia Bulletin. 2006: 32: 341-351. DOI: 10.1093/schbul/sbj02

[27] Averbeck BB, Evans S, Chouhan V, Bristow E, Shergill SS. Mint: probabilistic learning and inference in schizophrenia. Schizophrenia Research. 2011; 127 (1–3): 115-122. DOI: 10.1016/j.schres.2010.08.009

[28] Lincoln TM, Ziegler M, Mehl S, Rief W. Mint: the jumping to conclusions bias in delusions: specificity and changeability. Journal of Abnormal Psychology. 2010; 119 (1): 40-49. DOI: 10.1037/a0018118

[29] Veckenstedt R, Randjbar S, Vitzthum F, Hottenrott B, Woodward TS, Moritz S. Mint: incorrigibility, jumping to conclusions and decision threshold in schizophrenia. Cognitive Neuropsychiatry. 2011; 16 (2): 174-192. DOI: 10.1080/13546805.2010.536084

[30] Moritz S, Woodward TS. Mint: plausibility judgment in schizophrenic patients: evidence for a liberal acceptance bias. German Journal of Psychiatry. 2004; 7: 66-74.

[31] Moritz S, Woodward TS, Hausmann D. Mint: incautious reasoning as a pathogenetic factor for the development of psychotic symptoms in schizophrenia. Schizophrenia Bulletin. 2006; 32: 327-331

[32] Moritz S, Woodward TS. Mint: a generalized bias against disconfirmatory evidence in schizophrenia. Psychiatry Research. 2006; 142: 157-165. DOI: 10.1016/j.psychres. 2005.08.016

[33] Munz MT. Mint: Jumping to Conclusions, Liberal Acceptance and the Bias Against18 Disconfirmatory Evidence: An Evaluation of Reasoning Deviations in Delusions. Rostock: Rostock University, 2011. DOI: urn:nbn:de:gbv:28-diss2012-0089-520

[34] Garety P, Freeman D. Mint: the past and future of delusion research: from the inexplicable to the treatable. Brain Journal Psychiatry. 2013; 203: 327-333.

[35] Kwapil TR, Barrantes Vidal N, Silvia PJ. Mint: the dimensional structure of the Wisconsin schizotypy scales: factor identification and construct validity. Schizophrenia Bulletin. 2008; 34: 444-457.

[36] Konings M, Back M, Hansen M, van Os J, Krabbendam L. Mint: validity and reability of the CAPE: a self-report instrument for the measurement of psychotic experiences in the general population. Acta Psychiatry Scand. 2006; 114 (1): 55-61.

[37] Evans SL, Averbeck BB, Furl N. Mint: jumping to conclusions in schizophrenia. Neuropsychiatric Disease and Treatment. 2015; 11: 1615-1624. DOI: 10.2147/ NDT.S56870

[38] Colbert SM, Peters ER. Mint: need for closure and jumping-to-conclusions in delusion-prone individuals. The Journal of Nervous and Mental Disease. 2002; 190 (1): 27-31.

[39] Kruglanski AW. Mint: the psychology of being "right": the problem of accuracy in social perception and cognition. Psychological Bulletin. 1989; 106: 395-409.

[40] Webster D, Kruglanski A. Mint: individual differences in need for cognitive closure. Journal of Personality and Social Psychology. 1994; 67: 1049-1062.

[41] Federico CM, Ergun D, Hunt CV. Mint: opposition to equality and support for tradition as mediators of the relationship between epistemic motivation and ideological affinity. Journal of Research in Personality. 2014; 17 (4): 524-541. DOI: 10.1177/1368430213517273

[42] Juárez Ramos V. Mint: Cognitive Neuroscience: Differences between different populations in decision making tasks. Granada: University of Granada; 2014.

[43] McKay R, Langdon R, Coltheart M. Mint: jumping to delusions? Paranoia, probabilistic reasoning and need for closure. Cognitive Neuropsychiatry. 2007; 12 (4): 362-376. DOI: 10.1080/13546800701203769

[44] Bentall RP, Swarbrick R. Mint: the best laid schemas of paranoid patients: autonomy, sociotropy and need for closure. Psychology and Psychotherapy. 2003; 76 (Pt 2): 163-171.

[45] Moritz S, Veckenstedt R, Hottenrott B, Woodward TS, Randjbar S, Lincoln TM. Mint: different sides of the same coin? Intercorrelations of Cognitive Biases in Schizophrenia. 2010; 15 (4): 406-421. DOI: 10.1080/13546800903399993

[46] Gaweda L, Moritz S, Kokoszka A. Impaired discrimination between imagined and performed actions in schizophrenia. Psychiatry Research. 2012; 195: 1-8. DOI: 0.1016/j.psychres.2011.07.035

[47] Peters MJ, Cima MJ, Smeets T, de Vos M, Jelicic M, Merckelbach H. Did I say that word or did you? Executive dysfunctions in schizophrenic patients affect memory efficiency, but not source attributions. Cognition Neuropsychiatry. 2007; 12: 391-411.

[48] Barber B. Odean T. Boys will be boys: gender, overconfidence and common stock investment, Quarterly Journal of Economics. 2001; 116: 261-292.

[49] Peters MJ, Hauschildt M, Moritz S, Jelinek L. Impact of emotionality on memory and meta-memory in schizophrenia using video sequences. Journal of Behavior Therapy and Experimental Psychiatry. 2013; 44 (1): 77-83. DOI: 10.1016/j.jbtep.2012.07.003

[50] Köther U, Veckenstedt R, Vitzthum F, Roesch-Ely D, Pfueller U, Scheu, F, Moritz, S. "Don't give me that look" — overconfidence in false mental state perception in schizophrenia. Psychiatry Research. 2012; 196: 1-8. DOI: http://dx.doi.org/10.1016/j.psychres.2012.03.004

Chapter 6

Circuits Regulating Pleasure and Happiness in Schizophrenia: The Neurobiological Mechanism of Delusions

Anton J.M. Loonen and Svetlana A. Ivanova

Additional information is available at the end of the chapter

http://dx.doi.org/10.5772/66412

Abstract

A recently developed model describes how evolutionary old neuronal systems allow free-moving animals, including humans, to escape from threats and discomfort and to acquire sufficient necessities to maintain life and to continue as a species. The amygdala has an essential role in regulating these fundamental reward-seeking and misery-fleeing behaviours. This is probably related to the ancient character of the corticoid and ganglionic parts of the amygdaloid complex. During evolution almost the entire ventral and lateral pallium (cortex) of the first vertebrates went up into the superficial and deep amygdalar nuclei, and their entire striatum and pallidum went up into the extended amygdala. An important role of the amygdala is selecting the sensory cues which are relevant for reward-seeking and misery-fleeing behaviour and should be paid attention to in order to increase the animal's chances. This corresponds to attentive salience. Disturbances of this process in humans may lead to delusions. It has been suggested that in patients with schizophrenia this aberrant salience results from dopaminergic hyperactivity. The authors of this chapter believe that aberrant salience can result from dysfunctions everywhere within the chain: neocortex, corticoid amygdala, hippocampal complex, medial septum, medial habenula, midbrain nuclei and ventral tegmental area.

Keywords: amygdala, hippocampus, habenula, salience, delusions, subcortical network

1. Introduction

Two basic principles of animal life are essential for survival of the individual and as a species. Firstly, the animal should be motivated to obtain food, warmth, sexual gratification and comfort. Secondly, the animal should be motivated to escape from predators, cold, sexual competitors and other forms of adversity. To survive as an individual and a species, even our oldest ocean-dwelling ancestors living over 560 million years ago must have been able to react to the environment to feed, evade predators, defend territory and reproduce. Hence, their primitive nervous systems must have regulated the necessary behaviours and incorporated the most essential structures of all today's freely moving Animalia. However, since then the human brain passed through a long evolutionary pathway during which particularly the forebrain showed major changes. The earliest vertebrate brain almost completely lacked the forerunner of the human neocortex and the dorsal parts of the basal ganglia [1, 2]. These newer parts of the brain are believed to determine human behaviour to a high degree and consequently receive most attention in research of processes explaining the genesis of mental disorders (see, e.g. Ref. [3]). This contrasts the involvement in psychic disorders of those behavioural processes described above as also being displayed by the most primitive vertebrates. We want to suggest that these actions are still regulated in humans by brain structures derived from the primitive forebrain of the earliest vertebrates. Therefore, we described the anatomy of the forebrain of the earliest human vertebrate ancestors, which is believed to be comparable with the brain of lampreys [2]. From a comparison of the striatum of lampreys to that of anuran amphibians and younger vertebrates, it can be concluded that the striatum of lampreys is the forerunner of the human nuclear amygdala [4]. In anuran amphibians (frogs and toads), the lamprey's striatum is retrieved as central and medial amygdaloid nuclei, while a later ventral striatum for the first time appears in its direct vicinity [2, 4]. The lamprey's forebrain also contains a structure of which the connections are very well conserved in more recent human ancestors: the habenula. The habenula constitutes—together with the stria medullaris and pineal gland—the epithalamus and consists of medial and lateral parts [5]. The habenula regulates the intensity of reward-seeking and misery-fleeing behaviour probably in all our vertebrate ancestors. In lampreys the activity of the habenula is in turn regulated by a specific structure: the habenula-projecting globus pallidus. It is tempting to speculate that this structure has a similar role in humans, but a clear anatomical human equivalent with the same function has not yet been identified. Based upon the evolution of the basal ganglia in vertebrates and the mechanism of the emotional response, we postulate the existence of two systems regulating the intensity of the aforementioned behaviours [6, 7]. These two circuits include the activities of extrapyramidal and limbic basal ganglia and are collaborating in a yin-and-yang-like fashion. The two basal ganglia systems are linked together by the core and shell parts of the nucleus accumbens (NAcb), which regulates motivation to show reward-seeking and misery-fleeing behaviour, respectively.

The amygdala is believed to address the ability of learning to value sensory information (attentive salience). This capacity is essential to determine which sensory information is of vital importance to react on with reward-seeking or misery-fleeing behaviour. Aberrant salience is believed to be a crucial component of the mechanism of (schizophrenic) psychosis and the antipsychotic effects of dopamine antagonists [8]. We believe that the amygdala regulates the behavioural output by affecting the connection of the ancient forebrain (amygdala, hippocampus) with the monoaminergic centres of the midbrain through the

http://dx.doi.org/10.5772/66412

medial and lateral habenula. Therefore, we will describe the evolution of the amygdaloid complex and its final anatomy and functioning. Subsequently, we will integrate these findings with our model of neuronal circuits regulating pleasure and happiness and give an explanation how the connection between amygdala and habenula is involved regulating these behaviours.

2. Evolution of the amygdaloid complex in vertebrates

An important reason for us to become interested in the embryology, connectivity and neuroanatomy of primitive vertebrates is the scientific notion that their primitive brains may reflect earlier evolutionary stages of the current human brain. Hence, the brains of lampreys, sharks, lungfishes, frogs, turtles, opossums, rats and monkeys correspond to the brains of human ancestors from about 560 million years ago until now [9]. The very first vertebrate is supposed to be an animal comparable with modern lamprey [2]. This animal has a head containing a brain and it has vertebrates, but not yet a lower jaw. The lamprey forebrain consists of olfactory bulbs, medial and lateral pallium, subpallium and diencephalon (extensive thalamus). The lateral pallium already forms a primitive hemisphere (**Figure 1**). However, some controversy exists how to divide it into different fields. The question emerges whether the lamprey has a dorsal pallium, a structure which gives rise to the majority of the neocortex in mammals. We have concluded that our earliest vertebrate ancestor (comparable with lamprey) must already have had a dorsal pallium, but it functions as an extension of the medial pallium. Lamprey medial pallium is considered to give rise to the hippocampal complex in tetrapods [10]. The ventral pallium which appears to be present in all vertebrates, but also in hagfishes, is related to olfactory structures. It is included as part of the amygdala in tetrapods [10].

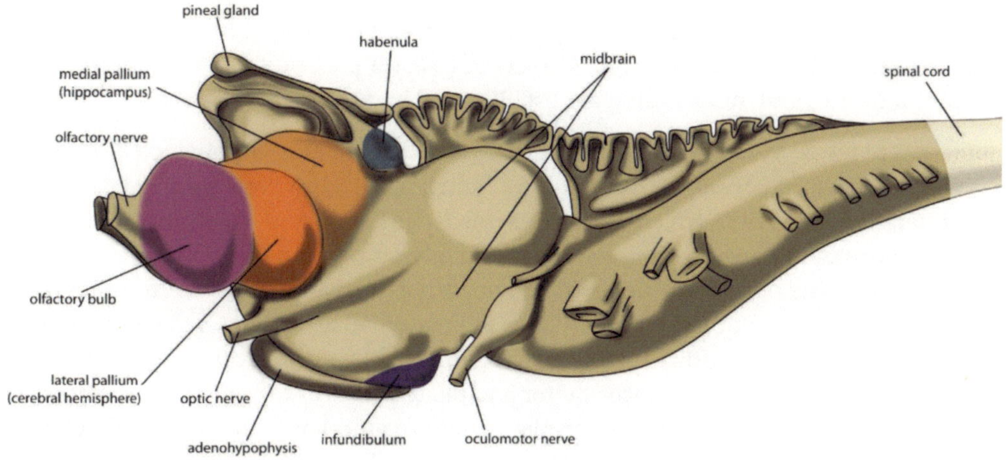

Figure 1. Central nervous system of lamprey.

2.1. Evolution of the cerebral cortex

Studying the development of the human cerebral cortex during subsequent steps of evolution brings a few typical problems. Firstly, in reptiles and birds, the neocortex developed in another direction than in mammals [10]. Secondly, a large part of the cerebral cortex in mammals is laminated (organised in three or six different layers), while the pallium in non-mammals is primary organised in a non-laminar fashion. However, by integrating comparative neuroanatomy with comparative embryology and developmental genetics, a clear picture can be created on the evolutionary development of human cerebral cortex [10–12].

In human embryos the future insula is the first 'neo'cortical structure to develop [13, 14]. The primordial insula is initially located on the free lateral surface of the cerebral hemisphere and adjoining the cortical amygdaloid regions on one side and olfactory cortical regions on the other [13, 15]. This is highly comparable to the position of the dorsal pallium in lamprey hemispheres [16]. According to the von Baerian theory, embryos of later-descendent species resemble the embryos of earlier-descendant species to the point of their divergence. So, it may be concluded that the human insula is the most ancient part of the neocortex. In addition, the lamprey has a small but well-developed dorsal thalamus (the part forming the proper so-called thalamus in humans), which connects the tectum (e.g. somatosensory and viscerosensory information) and optic tract (visual information) with caudal parts of the pallium (mainly hippocampal primordium and subhippocampal lobe, i.e. medial pallium) [17].

In amphibians, the dorsal pallium has significantly expanded in comparison to lamprey dorsal pallium, and it covers almost the entire roof of the hemisphere in these animals [18]. Fibres of neurons within these dorsal pallial fields run ipsilaterally to other pallial regions (medial, lateral, ventral), to the septum and to the amphibian striatopallidum [18]. However, fibres running from the thalamus to the primitive cerebral cortex are certainly not restricted to the newly present dorsal fields [19–21]. Anterior parts of the anuran thalamus are projecting widely within the forebrain, while, e.g. visual information is also projected to the hypothalamus and brainstem [19]. From electrical recording and anatomical labelling experiments, it can be concluded that the anuran dorsal pallium does not yet has achieved its human input processing and output generating role [19–21] but is still part of a more extensive 'limbic' behavioural control system including almost all pallial and subpallial regions.

In more recent jawed vertebrates, the input to the dorsal thalamus largely increases and this leads to a significant expansion of the dorsal pallium [22, 23]. However, this expansion occurs along different lines in non-synapsid (reptiles, birds) and synapsid (mammals) animals [12, 23]. Both groups derive from a common sauropsid ancestor with a turtle-like brain. The dorsal thalamus consists of two divisions called lemnothalamus and collothalamus, dependent upon their brainstem input structures. Within the mammalian line, both thalamic divisions with their corresponding cortical fields developed [23]. These cortical fields comprise the subicular, cingulate, prefrontal, sensorimotor and related cortices of mammals. The described expansion resulted probably in a total displacement of ventral and medial pallial fields. The medial pallium became hippocampus and the ventral pallium became the most caudal edge of the frontal lobe (including olfactory tubercle) and cortical regions of the amygdaloid complex in the temporal lobe.

Secondary to the described synapsid development of the dorsal pallium, lamination of the cerebral cortex occurred [10, 24]. This lamination is absent in non-mammals and not restricted to new, originally dorsal, pallial fields [10]. Due to this lamination, the human neocortex consists of horizontal layers, intersected by vertical (or radial) columns that are stereotypically interconnected in the vertical dimension and comprise processing units [24, 25]. The expansion and elaboration of the cerebral neocortex during evolutionary development from primitive mammals to humans resulted in formation of new areas with new connections creating numerous extensive networks regulating different new or more sophisticated types of behaviour [24]. However, the majority of this progress is of relatively recent date.

2.2. Evolution of subcortical structures

The lamprey telencephalon can be divided into a dorsal, pallial region and a ventral, subpallial region. This subpallial part largely consists from the striatum, septum and preoptic area [17]. Sten Grillner and collaborators have demonstrated that the complete basal ganglia circuitry is already present in these phylogenetically oldest vertebrates [26, 27]. Moreover, these animals possess a subpallial structure (**Figure 2**), the habenula-projecting globus pallidus (GPh), which has an essential role in selecting behaviours that are either rewarding and should be continued or are not rewarding and should be abandoned [28]. We have hypothesised that lamprey striatal subpallium is included in nuclear amygdala of mammals [2]. However, some controversy exists concerning the fate of the GPh in more recent vertebrates. Lamprey also

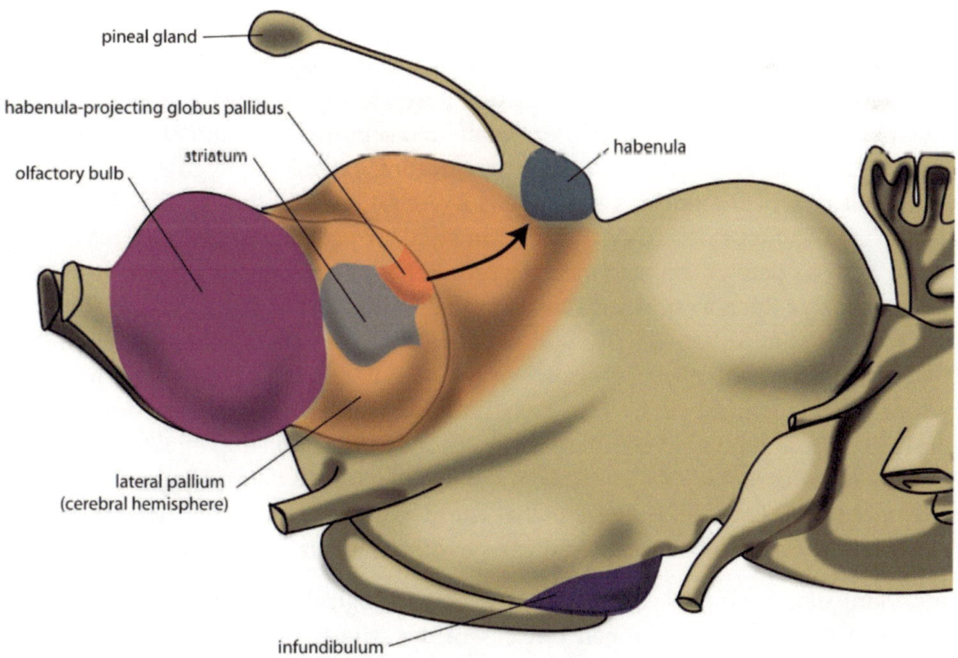

Figure 2. Position of the striatum and habenula-projecting globus pallidus of lamprey.

have an epithalamus which is very similar to its homologue in more modern animals [2]. This includes the output structures of the habenula via fasciculus retroflexus to midbrain nuclei.

It was formerly believed that the forebrain (especially its basal ganglia) underwent important changes during the evolution from anamniotes (lampreys, fishes, amphibians) to amniotes (reptiles, birds and mammals). However, the organisation of the basal ganglia is more conserved than previously thought [29]. The two main components of the basal ganglia develop embryologically from two different areas: the lateral ganglionic eminence (giving rise to the striatum) and the medial ganglionic eminence (giving rise to the pallidum). During embryological development different genes are brought to expression in order to regulate the regionalisation of these two areas. In particular, the transcription factor Nkx2.1 is expressed in the medial ganglionic eminence (and not the lateral one), and the expression of this gene in combination with that of others has been used to characterise pallidal basal ganglia in embryos of amniotes and anamniotes [29]. These authors were able to identify striatal and pallidal regions in cartilaginous fishes, ray-finned fishes, lungfishes and amphibians. However, in the subpallium of lampreys, a pallidal region could not be identified because these animals lack an Nkx2.1-expressing zone. Therefore, it was suggested that the pallidum is still absent in agnathans and first appeared during or after the transition from jawless to jawed vertebrates [30]. However, since Stephenson-Jones and colleagues [26, 27] have demonstrated the existence of a complete extrapyramidal circuitry in the subpallium of lamprey, this proposal of Moreno and co-workers [30] has to be rejected. In lampreys pallidal structures do exist in spite of the absence of expression of Nkx2.1 during the embryonic development of this structure.

The nuclear part of the amygdaloid complex is another derivative of the lateral ganglionic eminence, and the development of the amphibian amygdaloid complex has been studied in detail by Moreno and González [4, 31–33]. Within the anuran forebrain, the striatum (anterior) is continuous with the central and medial amygdala (posterior) and clearly separated from pallidum, bed nucleus of the stria terminalis and septum [4]. In humans, the bed nucleus of the stria terminalis is continuous with the connecting extended amygdala on one side and with the shell part of the nucleus accumbens (NAcbS) on the other [2, 25]. As a matter of fact, the original concept described the centromedial amygdala and bed nucleus of the stria terminalis both as part of the extended amygdala [34]. The investigations made clear that the organisation of the ancestral tetrapod (amphibian-like) amygdaloid complex is retained within more recent ancestors [35]. Evolution of the anamnio-amniotic (mammalian) striatum probably occurred in a modular sense when a more lateral part of the striatum was added every time when a cortical part with a new function was added to the expanding the neocortex [1, 36]. The amygdaloid complex derives from pallial and subpallial territories. Pallial (corticoid) structures include the cortical amygdala (olfactory and vomeronasal) and the basolateral complex deep to it [37]. These pallial components originate from lateral and ventral pallial regions and are also maintained during evolution of amniotic vertebrates [35, 37].

An important discovery during studying the embryological development of anuran basal ganglia was the finding that the bed nucleus of the stria terminalis (BST) and part of the septum are also of pallidal instead of striatal origin [29, 38]. This is interesting because the BST is a suitable structure to execute the functions of the limbic component of lamprey

http://dx.doi.org/10.5772/66412

habenula-projecting globus pallidus. The architecture and connectivity of the rat BST has been studied in detail by Larry Swanson and collaborators. It becomes evident that the BST is an extremely complex set of nuclei, which can be separated into dorsal, lateral and ventral areas [39]. These nuclei receive input from the central amygdaloid nucleus (innervating various parts of the anterior BST division) and medial amygdaloid nucleus (preferentially innervating the posterior BST division), but not from the superficial and deep corticoid nuclei of the amygdala [40]. It is concluded that BST is a rostral differentiation of the pallidum receiving massive GABAergic input from centromedial amygdala and giving again GABAergic output to brainstem motor systems and thalamocortical re-entrant loops [40]. Viewed broadly, BST posterior division cell groups share massive bidirectional connections with the medial amygdaloid nucleus and other amygdaloid components of the accessory olfactory system, and they send massive projections to hypothalamic control centres regulating reproduction and defence [41]. The BST anterolateral group projects to the ventral autonomic control network, to midbrain structures modulating the expression of orofacial and locomotor somatosensory responses and to the ventral striatopallidal system. This suggests that the anterolateral group is primary involved in appetitive feeding (eating and drinking) behaviour [41]. The lateral habenula hardly receives any fibres from these BST areas. However, the anteromedial BST division projects to the lateral habenula [41, 42]. In our opinion, it is very well possible that the anteromedial division of the rat BST contains glutamatergic neurons which are running to the lateral habenula and have similar function as lamprey GPh neurons. Moreover, the anterior BST division receives input from hippocampus (ventral subiculum) and infralimbic cortex (comparable with the human subgenual anterior cingulate cortex, Brodmann area 25 (BA25)). This connectivity probably corresponds to the cortical input to the habenula-projecting globus pallidus.

2.3. Conclusion: evolution of the amygdaloid complex

The endbrain (telencephalon) of the very first vertebrates can be considered to be the evolutionary starting point of the human amygdaloid complex. Its pallium largely consisted of ventral, lateral and medial fields. Its dorsal pallium was not contributing to a very significant extent. Its subpallium contained a striatopallidal complex for motor control and a habenula-projecting globus pallidus for decision-making. During evolution to an amphibian-like ancestor, the dorsal pallium developed to a significant extent, but it can still be considered an extension of the medial pallium. This can be concluded from its connectivity with other pallial and subpallial structures as well as from its input received from the dorsal thalamus. The medial pallium later developed into the hippocampus. At a subpallidal level, the primitive striatopallidal complex becomes nuclear amygdala and bed nucleus of the stria terminalis, respectively. This limbic striatopallidal structure will later become the human extended amygdala of Heimer [34]. Next to the amygdaloid complex, a new ventral and dorsal striatopallidal complex arises in amphibians which will form the extrapyramidal system in our mammalian ancestors. In our opinion it actually took until the evolution of our mammalian ancestors before the dorsal pallium was actually transformed into the current neocortex. The massive growth of this neocortex resulted in a C-shaped and outside-inward curving of the cerebral hemispheres. The medial pallium became hippocampus and the ventral pallium superficial and deep corticoid amygdala. This means that almost the entire cerebral hemisphere is of quite recent origin. This is probably also true for the limbic cortical-subcorti-

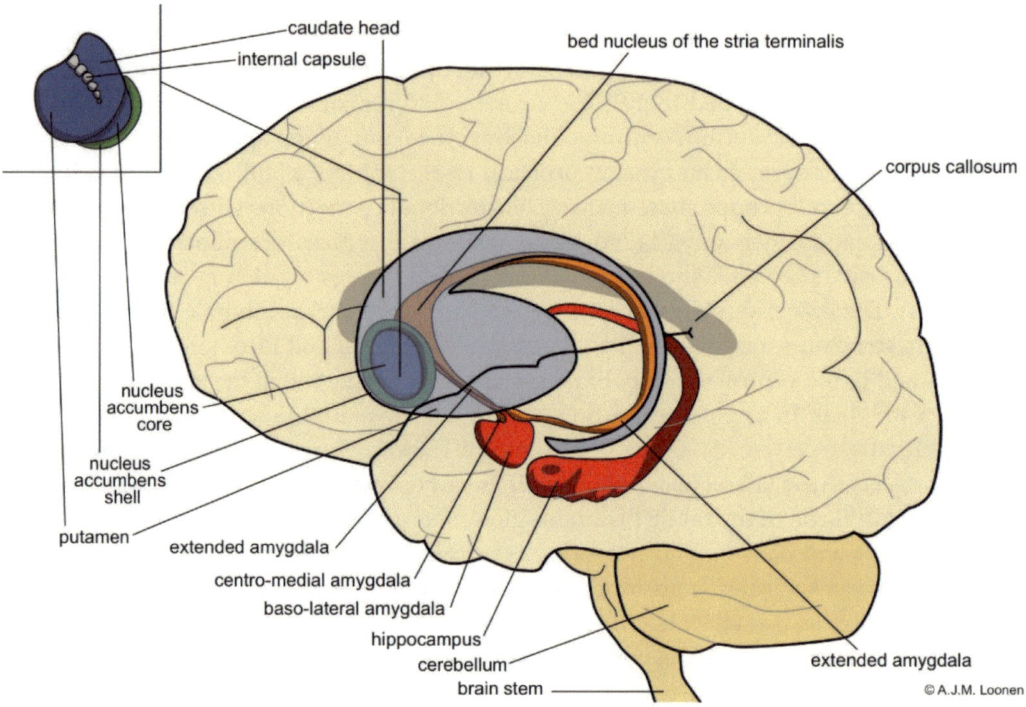

Figure 3. Position of the limbic basal ganglia (extended amygdala and nucleus accumbens shell) relative to the extrapyramidal striatum (caudate nucleus, putamen, nucleus accumbens core) and hippocampus.

cal-cortical connectivity we have previously suggested [2, 6]. Corticoid amygdaloid output reaches the hypothalamus and brainstem (to minor extent directly and) largely along nuclear amygdala (striatal amygdala) and bed nucleus of the stria terminalis (pallidal amygdala). This directly results from the regulation of vegetative and motor behaviour by the striatum instead of the pallium in lamprey [2]. However, the human frontal neocortex is reached through connectivity with the dorsal thalamus. This last connectivity must have developed later during the evolution of the mammalian forebrain. The amygdaloid equivalent of the habenula-projecting globus pallidus is probably localised within the bed nucleus of the stria terminalis.

The final picture of the position of the human limbic and extrapyramidal basal ganglia is given in **Figure 3**.

3. Connectivity of the amygdaloid complex

The amygdaloid complex is a heterogeneous group of 13 nuclei and cortical areas located in the medial temporal lobe just rostral to the hippocampal formation [43]. The complex can

http://dx.doi.org/10.5772/66412

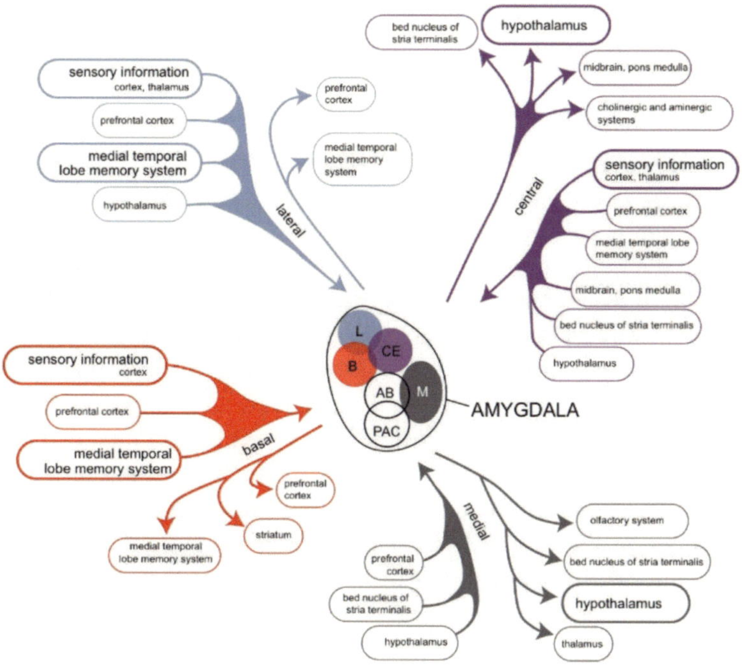

Figure 4. Overview of the connectivity of the rat amygdaloid complex [adapted from Ref. [45] with permission of the author].

neuroanatomically be divided into 'deep nuclei', 'superficial nuclei' and 'remaining nuclei' [43]. Both the cortical amygdalar nuclei and the basolateral amygdalar nuclear complex, which is located deep to it, have cortex-like cell types [44]. In contrast, the so-called extended amygdalar nuclei contain predominantly GABAergic spiny projection neurons, like the striatum [44]. In order to simplify, we usually divide the amygdala in a corticoid basolateral and a nuclear centromedial part (**Figure 3**). Each nucleus of the amygdala has a characteristic set of interconnections with other amygdalar nuclei and extrinsic brain regions (**Figure 4**) [43, 45]. Within the amygdalar nuclear complex, the primary flow is from corticoid to nuclear structures [46].

An unambiguous description of the structure and connectivity of the human amygdaloid amygdala is hampered by the existence of a predominance of contradictory, confusing, and unsubstantiated viewpoints both in recent and old scientific literature [47–49]. Moreover, the connections of the amygdaloid complex have been studied in mammalian animal species (mainly rats, cats and monkeys), which differ with respect to the extensiveness of their neocortex [48]. This large size of the neocortex causes dominance of projections from and to neocortical areas. Again looking into the connectivity of putative homologues of the amygdaloid complex in our early vertebrate ancestors may be of help. In amphibians, the amygdaloid complex is divided into three components: the vomeronasal amygdala, the olfactory/multimodal amygdala and the autonomic amygdala [4]. It should be realised that anuran species probably do not possess a true homologue of the human neocortex yet (see above). However, the anterior, lateral and medial areas of the anuran amygdaloid complex reveal connectivity which is roughly running ahead of the connectivity of the neocortex associated with amygdaloid complex [4, 50]. This includes output of the later deep corticoid and medial amygdaloid nucleus to the medial pallium, which is the later hippocampus.

Based on these start points, three or four components of amygdaloid connectivity can be distinguished: the accessory olfactory division, the main olfactory division, the autonomic division and the frontotemporal division [47, 48]. As possession of a true vomeronasal organ, which is originally the main source of input to the accessory olfactory division, by humans is still controversial, the first two may be added together in humans. The frontotemporal division is often primarily associated with strong bidirectional interactions with the prefrontal cortex and hippocampal formation [45, 46], but the amygdalo-hippocampal system can also be considered to be an output channel of the amygdaloid complex. The connectivity of the deep corticoid amygdaloid complex from and to the hippocampal complex is mediated through parahippocampal regions [51]. Via the fornix the hippocampus sends a GABAergic connection to the medial septum and a glutamatergic connection to the lateral septum [52, 53]. Reciprocally, cholinergic and to a far less extent GABAergic and glutamatergic fibres coming from the medial septum-diagonal band of Broca complex run through the fornix to the hippocampus [52, 53].

The four divisions of the amygdaloid system have more conjoined than separated functional significance. All regulate in combination with each other several components of instinctive, emotional behaviour. The accessory olfactory component is perhaps somewhat more involved in social behaviour related to reproduction and the autonomic part somewhat more with the regulation of visceral aspects of the emotional response. However, the abundancy of the interactions between separate amygdaloid areas and the extensive mixed connectivity with other brain structures [43–45] make that separate pathways cannot be clearly distinguished. An important part of this amygdaloid output is delivered, either directly or via hippocampus indirectly, to hypothalamic structures regulating reward-gaining and misery-fleeing behaviour [6, 54, 55]. These hypothalamic areas are also reached via the non-centromedial parts of the extended amygdala (including the bed nucleus of the stria terminalis) [49, 56]. However, a major role is played by the deep corticoid complex (mainly basolateral nuclei) in bidirectional interaction with prefrontal cortical areas, the hippocampal complex, as well as sensory cortical areas [44, 46, 57–59]. An essential characteristic of this bidirectional amygdaloid connectivity is the capability to learn from experiences through associative learning, complex response conditioning, episodic memorisation and so on [46]. The best description of the function of the amygdaloid complex is to analyse the complex input concerning the actual daily life situation within the individual's biotope (nature, flora, fauna, social circumstances) and to select the sensory input which deserves more attention in order to improve the current chances (misery fleeing and reward seeking). The amygdala also receives information about the environment from the sensory thalamus and sensory cortices. The input is compared with memorised information and modulated by programmes concerning implicit and explicit behavioural output. This includes direct inhibition of the amygdala-dependent emotional response when this is expected to be more profitable. This last function is primarily attributed to ventromedial areas of the prefrontal cortex [6, 60, 61]. Traditionally, the amygdala is supposed to

http://dx.doi.org/10.5772/66412

induce an emotional response mainly by giving output to the hypothalamus and brainstem via the centromedial nucleus after this validation process has been completed [46]. We want to suggest that the significant part of output is additionally given via the hippocampus and fornix to medial and lateral septal areas [52, 53]. After comparison with memorised experiences in the hippocampus and processing within the septal area, this information may reach the medial habenula (MHb). The septum, particularly the medial septum and the adjacent nucleus of the diagonal band of Broca, is the main input to the MHb [5, 62, 63]. Although the MHb has been far less extensively studied than the lateral habenula (LHb), experimental data support hyperactivity of the MHb to be associated with depression, anxiety and fear [63]. The MHb projects through the inner area of the fasciculus retroflexus to the interpeduncular nucleus within the midbrain [5, 62, 64, 65]. The interpeduncular nucleus is a singular, unpaired structure located at the ventral midline of the midbrain [62, 66]. The major efferent pathways originating in the interpeduncular nucleus project to the dorsal tegmental nucleus [66], the ventral tegmental area [62] and the raphe nuclei [62, 64]. However, the interpeduncular nucleus is well known for its widespread projections both ascending and descending [62, 66]. Hence, the above pathway from the corticoid amygdala, via hippocampus, septal nuclei, medial habenula and interpeduncular nucleus to ventral tegmental area and raphe nuclei, may represent a primary regulation mechanism to increase or decrease the intensity of the emotional misery-fleeing response.

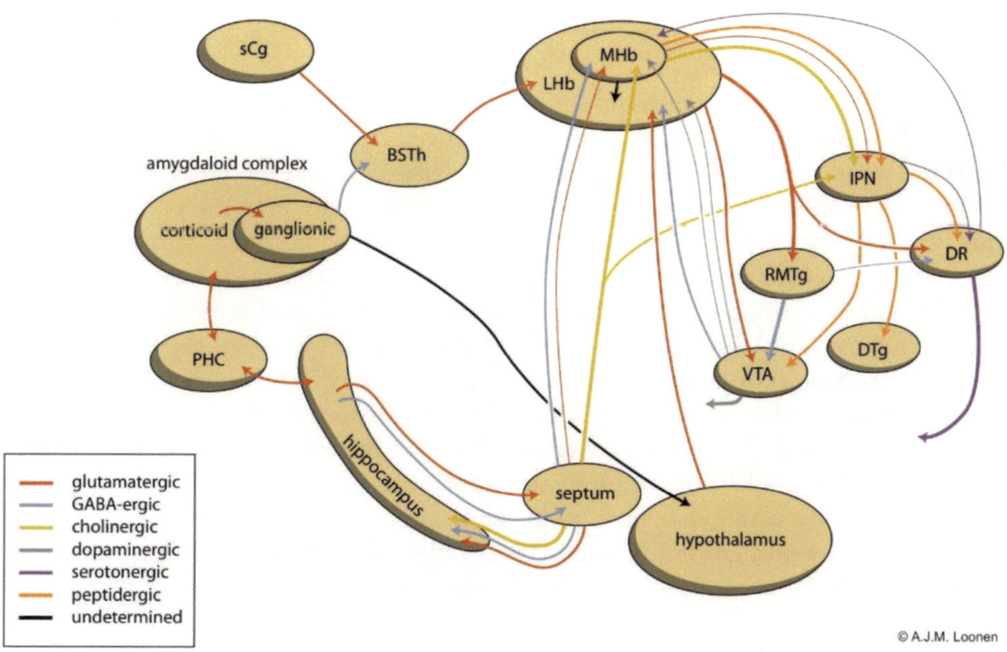

Figure 5. Scheme showing the connectivity of limbic (cortical) system to the midbrain through the habenular complex. BSTh, habenula-projecting part of the bed nucleus of the stria terminalis; DR, dorsal raphe nucleus; DTg, dorsal tegmental nucleus; IPN, interpeduncular nucleus; LHb, lateral habenula; MHb, medial habenula; PHC, parahippocampal cortex; RMTg, rostromedial tegmental nucleus; sCg, subgenual cingulate gyrus; and VTA, ventral tegmental area.

In addition, the amygdala affects the activity of the ventral tegmental area through a pathway including the lateral habenula. We want to suggest that anteromedial division of the bed nucleus of the stria terminalis contains the human limbic equivalent of the lamprey habenula-projecting globus pallidus (GPh). This area receives input from GABAergic projection neurons originating within the central amygdaloid nucleus [40] and gives output to medial and caudal regions of the lateral habenula [41, 42]. When this limbic GPh is functioning similar to lamprey GPh, the amygdala can inhibit reward-seeking behaviour by stimulating the pathway, which runs from corticoid amygdala, through central amygdala, anteromedial bed nucleus of the stria terminalis, lateral habenula and rostromedial tegmental nucleus to ventral tegmental area (**Figure 5**).

In conclusion, the amygdaloid complex plays an essential role in fear and anger control, perception and attention to relevant sensory input (including, e.g. facial expression in order to allow adequate social functioning), by validating this input with respect to their significance for reward-seeking and misery-fleeing behaviour. The activity of this emotional response is regulated through a pathway including the habenula, in which two routes can be distinguished: one including the hippocampus, septal nuclei and medial habenula and the other including central amygdala, bed nucleus of the stria terminalis and lateral habenula.

4. A model for the regulation of pleasure and happiness

4.1. Cortical regulation of behaviour

Behaviour can be considered a mechanism where the brain manages input to create a specific output, which enables the organism to adapt to changed circumstances within the biosphere. In humans, input from the senses is primarily translated within the cerebral cortex into a specific behavioural output. Sensory information is processed within the posterior cerebral cortex in a stepwise fashion [25, 67]. Specific information is integrated with other sensory information and transmitted from the primary sensory cortex to the secondary sensory cortex, from there to the association cortex and so on. Within the anterior cerebral cortex, a similar now diverging flow of information occurs, which leads to the activation of specific brain regions, e.g. the motor cortex. Apart from this stepwise analysis, other fibres connect to more distant regions that run in parallel. Every neural connection is capable of learning, due to the characteristics of glutamatergic transmission, which can increase or decrease the sensitivity of connecting synapses by inducing long-term potentiation (LTP) or long-term depression (LTD). Therefore, the cortex can 'learn' to transmit specific sensory information to a specific output unit via a 'preferred' cortical tract. Accordingly, the cerebral cortex learns to interpret sensory information and produce a specific behavioural response.

4.2. Subcortical regulation of behaviour

Although this process is expedient, it can be expected to be highly sensitive to dysregulation, both in routine functions and in learning. Therefore, a parallel circuit has evolved, which includes subcortical structures. All processing units in the cerebral cortex also send information to the

http://dx.doi.org/10.5772/66412

basal ganglia [68]. The route through the basal ganglia and thalamus leads to corresponding processing units in the anterior cortex [69]. This parallel circuit has stimulatory and inhibitory pathways, and its glutamatergic synapses can also induce LTP and LTD. Therefore, this parallel route through the basal ganglia enables the brain to correct serially transmitted information, when it arrives at the 'final' destination. Moreover, the connection through the basal ganglia is convergent [69]. Hence, the processing units in the posterior and anterior cortices and their outputs converge within this subcortical circuit to the same output unit. Again, the 'learning' ability of glutamatergic synapses within this framework makes it possible to process a constantly varying input and produce very complex, sophisticated output patterns, in a reproducible, precise fashion.

This organisation of connections is well known as the extrapyramidal system, which regulates cognition and movements [70]. In our mental function model, we suggest that a similar organisation can be distinguished within the limbic cortex, although here, the structure is more complex and less modular, due to the ancient origins of these structures. To simplify, we propose the corticoid regions of the amygdala to represent the primary limbic cortex. These corticoid regions are connected with many other cortical areas. The superficial (cortical) and deep (basolateral) corticoid regions of the amygdaloid complex can be considered input areas, and the centromedial (ganglionic or nuclear) region can be considered the output area of the amygdaloid complex [46]. In the earliest vertebrate ancestors, the striatum directly manages autonomic and motor control centres in lower diencephalon and brainstem [2]. In the lamprey very limited connectivity exists between pallial (cortex) areas and diencephalic and brainstem control centres. This is also true within the corresponding system in mammals: only light connectivity has been found between corticoid amygdalar areas and the hypothalamus or brainstem [45]. The stria terminalis connects the 'striatal' centromedial amygdala with its corresponding pallidum (bed nucleus of the stria terminalis) and also directly with the hypothalamus and brainstem [45]. Although the majority of output from the limbic basal ganglia flows to the brainstem, also connectivity exists with the (dorsal) thalamus and cerebral cortex. This is true for the output of the bed nucleus of the stria terminalis [40, 49] and for the output of the hypothalamus, which is probably related to affect the motor output of higher vertebrates, including humans, by inducing the drive to seek food, warmth, comfort, etc., or to escape from pain, thirst, misery, etc. [55]. This finally results in a limbic cortical-subcortical circuit that is more complex, but nevertheless essentially similar, to the well-known extrapyramidal system, provided that one realises that the cerebral neocortex was included within the circuit on a later evolutionary moment (**Figure 6**).

Hence, two types of cortical-subcortical circuits may be distinguished: extrapyramidal and limbic circuits. These systems have different ganglionic relay stations: the extrapyramidal circuit includes the dorsal and ventral striatum, and the limbic circuit includes the extended amygdala (as defined in Ref. [34]). These circuits are linked to each other by means of the nucleus accumbens, which serves as an interface between the two circuits [71]. The core part belongs to the extrapyramidal and the shell parts more to the limbic circuit. The extrapyramidal circuit regulates rational, cognitively constructed, skilled behaviour, which is often goal oriented and includes decision-making. The limbic circuit regulates emotional (instinctive and automatic) behaviours, which are often defensive, and this regulation includes (attentive)

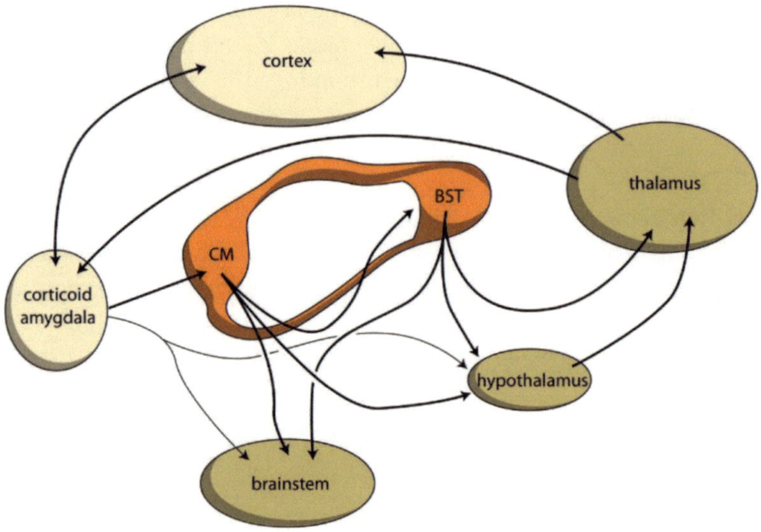

Figure 6. Limbic cortical-subcortical regulatory circuit. BST, bed nucleus of the stria terminalis; CM, centromedial amygdala; orange, extended amygdala; dark yellow, diencephalon and brainstem; and light yellow, corticoid amygdala and neocortex.

salience. The two systems influence each other in a reciprocal (yin-and-yang-like) fashion; moreover, both systems can inhibit or activate, as the situation demands. It is generally accepted that the prefrontal cortex (PFC) is in control of selecting the appropriate response [72, 73]. The dorsolateral PFC is particularly important for controlling rational responses, and the medial PFC controls emotional responses. Within the medial PFC, the orbitofrontal cortex (OFC) plays a particularly noteworthy role, because it is essential for regulating the direction of motivation [74].

4.3. Motivation to reward-seeking and misery-fleeing behaviour

Behaviour can be a reaction to an influence in the environment, or it can also be generated by the individual. To enable this proactive instead of reactive behaviour, motivation comes into play [73, 75]. Three stages of behavioural motivation can be distinguished: general motivation, initiative and selective precedence conveying (via inhibition). The OFC plays a significant role in regulating these processes by delivering input to the ventral striatum, the anterior cingulate cortex and the amygdala [74].

Although the extrapyramidal and limbic circuits regulate two different types of behaviour (constructed/rational and instinctive/intuitive, respectively), the individual must be highly motivated to express these conducts. This motivation requires the involvement of two specific structures: the NAcbC and the NAcbS (**Figure 7**) [71, 76, 77]. The NAcbC motivates the individual to show behaviour that may lead to a feeling of reward. The NAcbS motivates the individual to show behaviour that may lead to escape from adversity [6]. When high stimulation of these motivations suddenly ceases as its goal is obtained, the individual experiences feelings of pleasure (NAcbC) or feelings of happiness (NAcbS). Therefore, we dis-

http://dx.doi.org/10.5772/66412

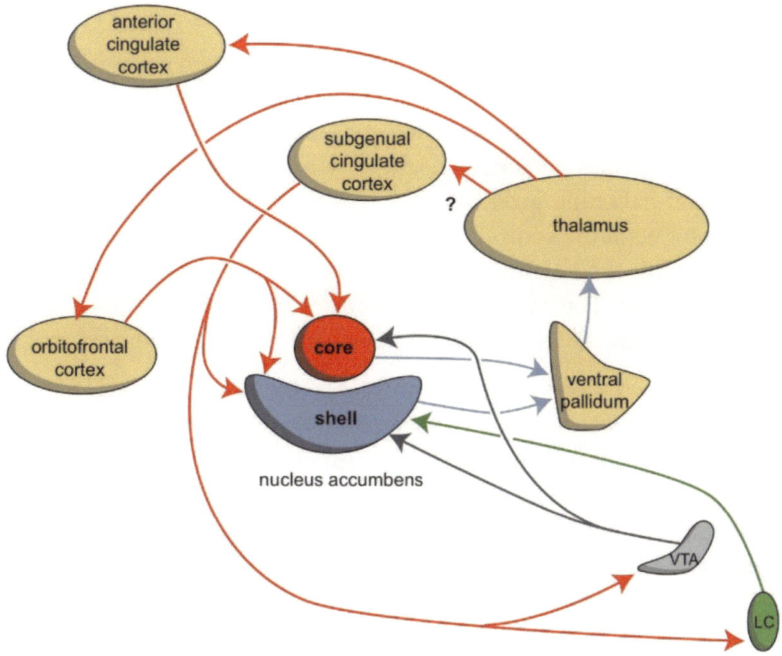

Figure 7. Stimulation of the core and shell of the nucleus accumbens (adapted from Ref. [76] with permission of the author). VTA, ventral tegmental area; LC, locus coeruleus. Red arrows, glutamatergic; blue arrows, GABAergic; grey arrows, dopaminergic; and green arrow, adrenergic.

tinguish between circuits that regulate pleasure and circuits that regulate happiness [6]. We have hypothesised that the best candidate for the perception of feelings of pleasure (reward) and happiness (euphoria) would be the insular cortex [7]. The posterior part of the insula contains areas for gustation, thermo-sensation, pain, somato-sensation and viscera-sensation [15]. Indeed, the insular cortex has been demonstrated to be involved in processing emotions like anger, fear, happiness, sadness or disgust and has been shown to display treatment-responsive changes of activity in different mood disorders [78].

4.4. Brainstem regulation of behaviour

The activities of the NAcbC and NAcbS, in turn, are regulated by monoaminergic nuclei within the midbrain. These nuclei transmit signals through dopaminergic (ventral tegmental area), adrenergic (norepinephrine, locus coeruleus) and serotonergic (raphe nuclei) tracts. In addition to their direct regulation of the NAcbC and/or NAcbS [6, 7], these monoaminergic nuclei regulate the activity of other, first relay station, basal ganglia and important parts of other areas in the forebrain. Therefore, it may be concluded that behavioural output is controlled at three levels within the brain. The highest level is the cerebral cortex (isocortex, limbic cortex, corticoid (cortical, basolateral) amygdala and hippocampal complex). The second level is the subcortical forebrain (dorsal striatum, ventral striatum, extended amygdala). The third level of control is the midbrain (monoaminergic regulation centres).

4.5. Habenular regulation of behaviour

As part of our model, we suggest that a fourth regulatory system exists, the habenula, which connects the cerebral cortex and midbrain systems (**Figure 8**) [6, 7]. Based on the regulation of appetitive behaviour in lampreys, we suggest the lateral habenula also to have an important regulatory function in humans [6]. In the lamprey, when a behaviour is particularly rewarding, the lateral habenula promotes this behaviour by intensifying stimulation of the phylogenetic homologue of the ventral tegmental area. However, when the reward is smaller than expected or absent, the behaviour is inhibited by affecting the ventral tegmental area equivalent of the lamprey. The medial habenula appears to play a similar role with respect to misery-fleeing behaviour as the lateral habenula with respect to reward-seeking activities.

The habenula belongs to the epithalamus, which also harbours the pineal gland and the stria medullaris. The habenula's projections to the midbrain were very well conserved during vertebrate evolution [7, 79], but its input structures are not so easily to be traced back from the anatomy of earlier vertebrates. The septum, particularly the medial septum and the adjacent nucleus of the diagonal band of Broca, is the main input structure of the medial habenula [5, 62, 63]. We suggest that by means of this pathway the corticoid amygdala (cortical and basolateral areas of the amygdaloid complex) gives input to the medial habenula (via hippocampal complex and fornix) (**Figure 5**). Although probably an important part of the functional

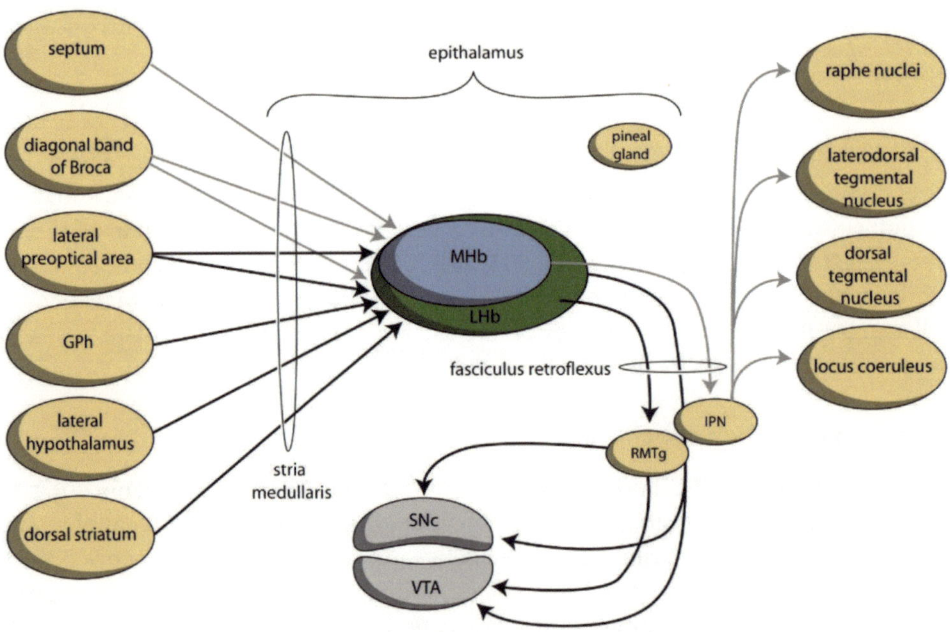

Figure 8. Simplified representation of the connectivity through the epithalamus (adapted with permission from Ref. [79]). GPh, habenula-projecting globus pallidus; IPN, interpeduncular nucleus; RMTg, rostromedial tegmental nucleus; SNc, substantia nigra, pars compacta; and VTA, ventral tegmental area. GPh depends upon the cortical-subcortical circuit being considered. GPh is localised within the bed nucleus of the stria terminalis in the limbic circuit, within the ventral pallidum concerning the motivational circuit and within the globus pallidus (border region, GPb) within the extrapyramidal circuit.

http://dx.doi.org/10.5772/66412

input to the lateral habenula has not yet been elucidated, this nucleus is known to receive excitatory input from the preoptic area, lateral hypothalamus and globus pallidus and from anterior cingulate and the medial prefrontal cortex [5, 80, 81]. Moreover, the lateral habenula also receives strong GABAergic innervations from various brain regions [82]. In addition, the medial habenula is directly giving input to the lateral habenula [83]. The striatopallidal (extended) amygdala is heavily (directly and indirectly) connected to the lateral hypothalamus. We suggest that the activity of the lateral habenula is modulated by this pathway. In addition, the bed nucleus of the stria terminalis contains the human equivalent of lamprey habenula-projecting globus pallidus, as we have argued above.

The corticoid amygdaloid complex is in a perfect position to increase the magnitude of misery-fleeing (happiness) over reward-seeking (pleasure) behaviour. This limbic cortex regulates the activity of monoaminergic centres within the midbrain by affecting the medial and lateral habenula. In addition, the amygdaloid complex regulates instinctive motivation to gain certain essential prerequisites to maintain life (such as food, water, warmth, etc.) by affecting the lateral hypothalamus.

4.6. Model for the regulation of behaviour

In conclusion, the extrapyramidal and limbic cortical systems regulate cognitive (rational) and instinctive behaviours, respectively. The intensity of behaviour that ultimately leads to reward is controlled by the cortico-striato-thalamo-cortical (CSTC) circuit that includes the NAcbC. The intensity of behaviour that ultimately leads to safety is controlled by the CSTC circuit that includes the NAcbS. On the temporal side of the brain, the amygdala determines

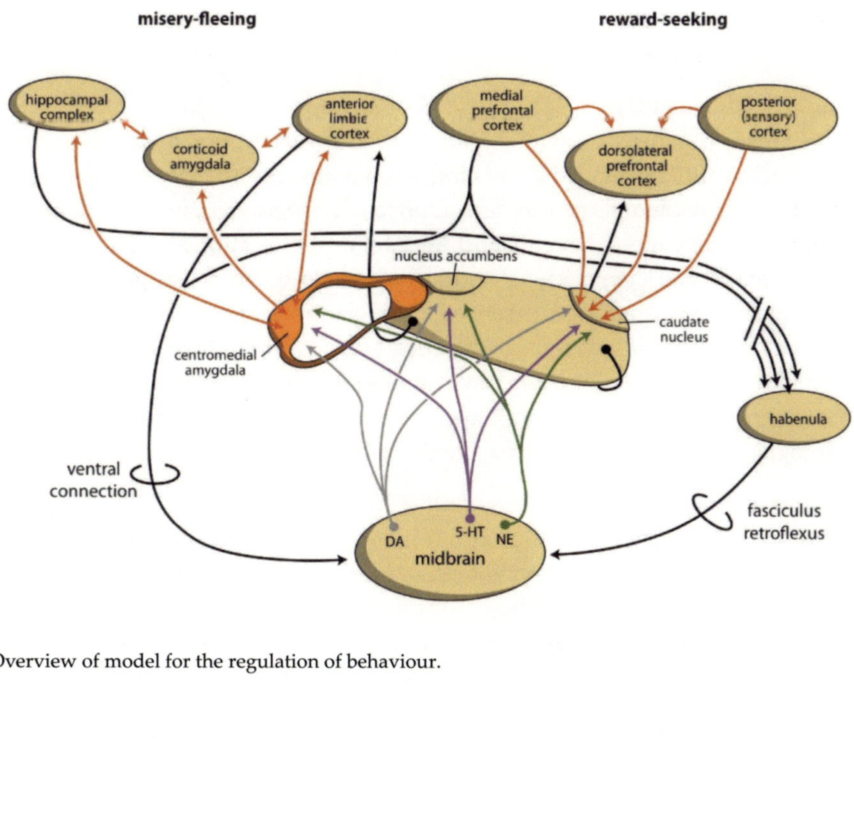

Figure 9. Overview of model for the regulation of behaviour.

the appropriateness of flight, fight, or appetitive responses. Based on attentive salience, it initiates the proper emotional component of behaviour. On the dorsal side of the brain, the caudate nucleus determines the suitability of the available repertoire of skilled behaviours; it selects the proper motor response to achieve the intended goals. The motivation to express these behaviours is regulated by monoaminergic centres within the midbrain. In turn, these monoaminergic centres are regulated by old and new parts of the cerebral cortex through a dorsal connection that travels through the medial and lateral habenula. Of note, the monoaminergic centres are also regulated by the medial prefrontal cortex via a direct ventral connection, which possibly travels through the medial forebrain bundle [7] (**Figure 9**).

5. From aberrant salience to schizophrenic psychosis

Salience attribution is the process of events and thoughts that come to grab attention, drive the actions and determine behaviour because of their associations with reward or punishment [84]. This corresponds very well to the role of the amygdaloid complex described in a few pages above: playing an essential role in fear and anger control by perception and paying attention to relevant sensory input (including, e.g. facial expression in order to allow adequate social functioning), by validating this input with respect to their significance for reward-seeking and misery-fleeing behaviour. As until mammals the neocortex was not capable of playing its input-processing and output-organising role as in humans, salience attribution was taken care of by the pallium of our anamniote and turtle-like ancestors. As described above this ancient pallium essentially corresponds with the superficial and deep corticoid amygdala and associated hippocampal areas. Later during evolution the interaction of the corticoid amygdala with neocortical areas became involved in the process, and in humans probably no part of the neocortex can be excluded from participating.

At the beginning of this century, Shitij Kapur [8, 85–88] proposed a model for the development of delusional systems in psychiatric disorders due to aberrant attribution of salience to objects and associations, which would normally be meaningless, but now are interpreted as being significant and to be dealt with considerable carefulness. Due to a dysregulated, hyperdopaminergic state this theory holds, environmental events and internal representations become associated with important elements of one's experiences and induce the creation of a cognitive construct (the delusion) to explain these strange occurrences. Hallucinations are believed to reflect the direct observation of these salient internal representations [85]. Antipsychotics decrease the salience of the abnormal experiences by blocking dopamine transmission and allow their resolution by making them unimportant. Howes and Kapur integrated vast experimental findings to this pathophysiological context of causing psychosis by inducing aberrant salience [88].

The model may correspond to the observation that delusions and hallucinations are not uncommon in the general population and not always result in a full-blown psychosis [89]. Substantial evidence suggests that psychotic-like experiences exist along a continuum in the general population [90]. Moreover, stress from life hassles can provoke delusional ideation [90]. In line with this, Jim van Os has suggested to replace the concept of schizophrenia being an illness with the model that it is a salience dysregulation syndrome [91–93].

An important limitation of the model is that the corticoid amygdala is integrated within at least four cortical networks regulating salience-involving processes [61, 84]. Within this context, especially, the interaction between the ventromedial prefrontal cortex and the corticoid amygdala may be essential. Therefore, the corticoid amygdala cannot be considered to be a separate salience-attributing structure, but is having this role in interaction with other cortical structures participating in the network [61].

6. Application of our model to explain the pathogenesis of schizophrenic psychosis

In our opinion, a weak point of Kapur's model is the starting point that the aberrant salience attribution is due to a dysregulated, hyperdopaminergic state. This is not necessarily true. Actually, the hyperdopaminergic state could result from dysregulation on every level within the corticoid amygdala to midbrain monoaminergic area chain, including input from neocortical areas to the corticoid amygdala and the influence of the habenula to relevant midbrain structures. In most psychotic disorders, the hyperdopaminergic state may not induce aberrant salience, but may result from it. This does not exclude that increased sensitivity to the effects of dopaminergic transmission may increase the vulnerability to become psychotic.

So, we propose that the primary dysregulation which causes psychotic symptoms in 'schizophrenia' is localised within the interaction between the corticoid amygdala, in interaction with neocortical fields, with midbrain monoaminergic centres. The ventromedial prefrontal cortex may be the principle pathway for the corticoid amygdala to interact with these other cortical areas. Via connections through the habenula, the amygdaloid complex regulates the activity of the midbrain monoaminergic centres which in turn regulate motivation to exhibit reward-seeking or misery-fleeing behaviour. Increased dopaminergic input to the basal ganglia may induce behavioural hyperactivity and to the parahippocampal region may lead to hallucinations [94]. The amygdaloid complex is also innervated with dopaminergic fibres. Dopamine may lead to increased sensitivity of the amygdala to induce an emotional response. Psychotic disorders may be due to increased dopaminergic activity within the amygdaloid complex, aberrant salience attribution due to genetic or learned (conditioned) neuronal faults or aberrant inhibition by the dorsomedial prefrontal cortex due to neurodegenerative network failure. However, the hyperdopaminergic state is probably not the essential factor causing schizophrenic psychosis, and this may explain why antidopaminergic agents, as are all current antipsychotic drugs, are not always effective in treating schizophrenic psychosis.

Acknowledgement

More anatomical details are provided with in Loonen AJM, Ivanova SA. Front Neurosci 2016;10:539. doi: 10.3389/fnins.2016.00539. Part of this work was supported by the Russian Science Foundation [Grant No. 14-15-00480].

Author details

Anton J.M. Loonen[1, 2*] and Svetlana A. Ivanova[3, 4]

*Address all correspondence to: a.j.m.loonen@rug.nl

1 Department of Pharmacy, University of Groningen, Groningen, The Netherlands

2 Mental Health Institute GGZ Westelijk Noord-Brabant, Halsteren, The Netherlands

3 Tomsk National Research Medical Center of the Russian Academy of Sciences, Mental Health Research Institute, Russian Federation

4 National Research Tomsk Polytechnic University, Tomsk, Russian Federation

References

[1] Robertson B, Kardamakis A, Capantini L, Pérez-Fernández J, Suryanarayana SM, Wallén P, Stephenson-Jones M, Grillner S. The lamprey blueprint of the mammalian nervous system. Prog Brain Res. 2014;212:337–49. doi: 10.1016/B978-0-444-63488-7.00016-1.

[2] Loonen AJM, Ivanova SA. Circuits regulating pleasure and happiness: the evolution of reward-seeking and misery-fleeing behavioral mechanisms in vertebrates. Front Neurosci. 2015;9:394. doi: 10.3389/fnins.2015.00394.

[3] Rolls ET. A non-reward attractor theory of depression. Neurosci Biobehav Rev. 2016;68:47–58. doi: 10.1016/j.neubiorev.2016.05.007.

[4] Moreno N, González A. The common organization of the amygdaloid complex in tetrapods: new concepts based on developmental, hodological and neurochemical data in anuran amphibians. Prog Neurobiol. 2006;78(2):61–90. doi: 10.1016/j.pneurobio.2005.12.005.

[5] Benarroch EE. Habenula: recently recognized functions and potential clinical relevance. Neurology. 2015;85(11):992–1000. doi: 10.1212/WNL.0000000000001937.

[6] Loonen AJM, Ivanova SA. Circuits regulating pleasure and happiness in major depression. Med Hypotheses. 2016;87(1):14–21. doi: 10.1016/j.mehy.2015.12.013.

[7] Loonen AJM, Schellekens AFA, Ivanova SA. Circuits regulating pleasure and happiness: a focus on addiction, beyond the ventral striatum. In: Meil WM, Ruby CL, eds. Recent advances in drug addiction research and clinical applications. Rijeka, Croatia: InTech, 2016; 1–20. doi: 10.5772/62707.

[8] Kapur S. How antipsychotics become anti-"psychotic" – from dopamine to salience to psychosis. Trends Pharmacol Sci. 2004;25(8):402–6. doi: 10.1016/j.tips.2004.06.005.

[9] Moreno N, González A. The non-evaginated secondary prosencephalon of vertebrates. Front Neuroanat. 2011;5:12. doi: 10.3389/fnana.2011.00012.

[10] Medina L, Abellán A. Development and evolution of the pallium. Semin Cell Dev Biol. 2009;20(6):698–711. doi: 10.1016/j.semcdb.2009.04.008.

[11] Butler AB, Reiner A, Karten HJ. Evolution of the amniote pallium and the origins of mammalian neocortex. Ann N Y Acad Sci. 2011;1225:14–27. doi: 10.1111/j.1749-6632.2011.06006.x.

[12] Montiel JF, Vasistha NA, Garcia-Moreno F, Molnár Z. From sauropsids to mammals and back: new approaches to comparative cortical development. J Comp Neurol. 2016;524(3):630–45. doi: 10.1002/cne.23871.

[13] O'Rahilly R, Müller F. The embryonic human brain. An atlas of developmental stages. Third edition. Hoboken, NJ: Wiley-Liss, 2006.

[14] Kalani MY, Kalani MA, Gwinn R, Keogh B, Tse VC. Embryological development of the human insula and its implications for the spread and resection of insular gliomas. Neurosurg Focus. 2009;27(2):E2. doi: 10.3171/2009.5.FOCUS0997.

[15] Nieuwenhuys R. The insular cortex: a review. Prog Brain Res. 2012;195:123–63. doi: 10.1016/B978-0-444-53860-4.00007-6.

[16] Ocaña FM, Suryanarayana SM, Saitoh K, Kardamakis AA, Capantini L, Robertson B, Grillner S. The lamprey pallium provides a blueprint of the mammalian motor projections from cortex. Curr Biol. 2015;25(4):413–23. doi: 10.1016/j.cub.2014.12.013.

[17] Nieuwenhuys R, Nicholson C. Chapter 10. Lampreys, Petromyzontoidea. In: Nieuwenhuys R, Ten Donkelaar HJ, Nicholson C, eds. The central nervous system of vertebrates. Berlin, Heidelberg: Springer-Verlag, 1998; 397–495.

[18] Roth G, Laberge F, Mühlenbrock-Lenter S, Grunwald W. Organization of the pallium in the fire-bellied toad *Bombina orientalis*. I: morphology and axonal projection pattern of neurons revealed by intracellular biocytin labeling. J Comp Neurol. 2007;501(3):443–64. doi: 10.1002/cne.21255.

[19] Roth G, Grunwald W, Dicke U. Morphology, axonal projection pattern, and responses to optic nerve stimulation of thalamic neurons in the fire-bellied toad *Bombina orientalis*. J Comp Neurol. 2003;461(1):91–110. doi: 10.1002/cne.10670.

[20] Laberge F, Roth G. Organization of the sensory input to the telencephalon in the fire-bellied toad, *Bombina orientalis*. J Comp Neurol. 2007;502(1):55–74. doi: 10.1002/cne.21297.

[21] Laberge F, Mühlenbrock-Lenter S, Dicke U, Roth G. Thalamo-telencephalic pathways in the fire-bellied toad *Bombina orientalis*. J Comp Neurol. 2008;508(5):806–23. doi: 10.1002/cne.21720.

[22] Butler AB. The evolution of the dorsal thalamus of jawed vertebrates, including mammals: cladistic analysis and a new hypothesis. Brain Res Brain Res Rev. 1994;19(1):29–65.

[23] Butler AB. The evolution of the dorsal pallium in the telencephalon of amniotes: cladistic analysis and a new hypothesis. Brain Res Brain Res Rev. 1994;19(1):66–101.

[24] Rakic P. Evolution of the neocortex: a perspective from developmental biology. Nat Rev Neurosci. 2009;10(10):724–35. doi: 10.1038/nrn2719.

[25] Loonen AJM. The mobile brain. The neuroscientific background of psychic functions Haarlem: Mension, 2013.

[26] Stephenson-Jones M, Samuelsson E, Ericsson J, Robertson B, Grillner S. Evolutionary conservation of the basal ganglia as a common vertebrate mechanism for action selection. Curr Biol. 2011;21(13):1081–91. doi: 10.1016/j.cub.2011.05.001.

[27] Stephenson-Jones M, Ericsson J, Robertson B, Grillner S. Evolution of the basal ganglia: dual-output pathways conserved throughout vertebrate phylogeny. J Comp Neurol. 2012;520(13):2957–73. doi: 10.1002/cne.23087.

[28] Stephenson-Jones M, Kardamakis AA, Robertson B, Grillner S. Independent circuits in the basal ganglia for the evaluation and selection of actions. Proc Natl Acad Sci U S A. 2013;110(38):E3670–9. doi: 10.1073/pnas.1314815110.

[29] González A, Morona R, Moreno N, Bandín S, López JM. Identification of striatal and pallidal regions in the subpallium of anamniotes. Brain Behav Evol. 2014;83(2):93–103. doi: 10.1159/000357754.

[30] Moreno N, González A, Rétaux S. Development and evolution of the subpallium. Semin Cell Dev Biol. 2009;20(6):735–43. doi: 10.1016/j.semcdb.2009.04.007.

[31] Moreno N, González A. Hodological characterization of the medial amygdala in anuran amphibians. J Comp Neurol. 2003;466(3):389–408. doi: 10.1002/cne.10887.

[32] Moreno N, González A. Localization and connectivity of the lateral amygdala in anuran amphibians. J Comp Neurol. 2004;479(2):130–48. doi: 10.1002/cne.20298.

[33] Moreno N, González A. Central amygdala in anuran amphibians: neurochemical organization and connectivity. J Comp Neurol. 2005;489(1):69–91. doi: 10.1002/cne.20611.

[34] Heimer L, Van Hoesen GW. The limbic lobe and its output channels: implications for emotional functions and adaptive behavior. Neurosci Biobehav Rev. 2006;30(2):126–47. doi: 10.1016/j.neubiorev.2005.06.006.

[35] Moreno N, González A. Evolution of the amygdaloid complex in vertebrates, with special reference to the anamnio-amniotic transition. J Anat. 2007;211:151–63. doi: 10.1111/j.1469-7580.2007.00780.x.

[36] Grillner S, Robertson B, Stephenson-Jones M. The evolutionary origin of the vertebrate basal ganglia and its role in action selection. J Physiol. 2013;591(22):5425–31. doi: 10.1113/jphysiol.2012.246660.

[37] Martínez-García F, Martínez-Marcos A, Lanuza E. The pallial amygdala of amniote vertebrates: evolution of the concept, evolution of the structure. Brain Res Bull. 2002;57(3–4):463–9. doi: 10.1016/S0361-9230(01)00665-7.

[38] Moreno N, Morona R, López JM, Domínguez L, Joven A, Bandín S, González A. Characterization of the bed nucleus of the stria terminalis in the forebrain of anuran amphibians. J Comp Neurol. 2012;520(2):330–63. doi: 10.1002/cne.22694.

[39] Ju G, Swanson LW. Studies on the cellular architecture of the bed nuclei of the stria terminalis in the rat: I. Cytoarchitecture. J Comp Neurol. 1989;280(4):587–602. doi: 10.1002/cne.902800409.

[40] Dong HW, Petrovich GD, Swanson LW. Topography of projections from amygdala to bed nuclei of the stria terminalis. Brain Res Brain Res Rev. 2001;38(1–2):192–246. doi: 10.1016/S0165-0173(01)00079-0.

[41] Dong HW, Swanson LW. Projections from bed nuclei of the stria terminalis, dorsomedial nucleus: implications for cerebral hemisphere integration of neuroendocrine, autonomic, and drinking responses. J Comp Neurol. 2006;494(1):75–107. doi: 10.1002/cne.20790.

[42] Dong HW, Swanson LW. Projections from bed nuclei of the stria terminalis, anteromedial area: cerebral hemisphere integration of neuroendocrine, autonomic, and behavioral aspects of energy balance. J Comp Neurol. 2006;494(1):142–78. doi: 10.1002/cne.20788.

[43] Freese JL, Amaral DG. Neuroanatomy of the primate amygdala. In: Whalen PJ, Phelps EA, eds. The human amygdala. New York: The Guilford Press, 2009; 3–42.

[44] McDonald AJ, Mott DD. Functional neuroanatomy of amygdalohippocampal interconnections and their role in learning and memory. J Neurosci Res. 2016. doi: 10.1002/jnr.23709. [Epub ahead of print].

[45] Pitkänen A. Connectivity of the rat amygdaloid complex. In: Aggleton JP, ed. The amygdala. A functional analysis. Oxford, UK: Oxford University Press, 2000; 31–115.

[46] Benarroch EE. The amygdala: functional organization and involvement in neurologic disorders. Neurology. 2015;84(3):313–24. doi: 10.1212/WNL.0000000000001171.

[47] Swanson LW, Petrovich GD. What is the amygdala?. Trends Neurosci. 1998;21(8):323–31 doi: 10.1016/S0166-2236(98)01265-X.

[48] Price JL. Comparative aspects of amygdala connectivity. Ann N Y Acad Sci. 2003;985:50–8. doi: 10.1111/j.1749-6632.2003.tb07070.x.

[49] Swanson LW. The amygdala and its place in the cerebral hemisphere. Ann N Y Acad Sci. 2003;985:174–84. doi: 10.1111/j.1749-6632.2003.tb07081.x.

[50] Roth G, Mühlenbrock-Lenter S, Grunwald W, Laberge F. Morphology and axonal projection pattern of neurons in the telencephalon of the fire-bellied toad *Bombina orientalis*: an anterograde, retrograde, and intracellular biocytin labeling study. J Comp Neurol. 2004;478(1):35–61. doi: 10.1002/cne.20265.

[51] Witter M. Chapter one: The parahippocampal region: past, present, and future. In: Witter M, Wouterlood F, eds. The parahippocampal region: organization and role in cognitive function. Oxford, UK: Oxford University Press, 2002; 3–19.

[52] Khakpai F, Nasehi M, Haeri-Rohani A, Eidi A, Zarrindast MR. Septo-hippocampo-septal loop and memory formation. Basic Clin Neurosci. 2013;4(1):5–23.

[53] Nieuwenhuys R, Voogd J, Van Huijzen C. 12 Telencephalon: hippocampus and related structures. In: The human central nervous system, Fourth edition. Berlin, Heidelberg: Springer, 2008; 361–400.

[54] Petrovich GD, Canteras NS, Swanson LW. Combinatorial amygdalar inputs to hippocampal domains and hypothalamic behavior systems. Brain Res Brain Res Rev. 2001;38(1–2):247–89.

[55] Sewards TV, Sewards MA. Representations of motivational drives in mesial cortex, medial thalamus, hypothalamus and midbrain. Brain Res Bull. 2003;61(1):25–49. doi: 10.1016/S0361-9230(03)00069-8.

[56] Waraczynski M. Toward a systems-oriented approach to the role of the extended amygdala in adaptive responding. Neurosci Biobehav Rev. 2016;68:177–94. doi: 10.1016/j.neubiorev.2016.05.015.

[57] Janak PH, Tye KM. From circuits to behaviour in the amygdala. Nature. 2015;517(7534):284–92. doi: 10.1038/nature14188.

[58] Wassum KM, Izquierdo A. The basolateral amygdala in reward learning and addiction. Neurosci Biobehav Rev. 2015;57:271–83. doi: 10.1016/j.neubiorev.2015.08.017.

[59] Rutishauser U, Mamelak AN, Adolphs R. The primate amygdala in social perception - insights from electrophysiological recordings and stimulation. Trends Neurosci. 2015;38(5):295–306. doi: 10.1016/j.tins.2015.03.001.

[60] Kim MJ, Loucks RA, Palmer AL, Brown AC, Solomon KM, Marchante AN, Whalen PJ. The structural and functional connectivity of the amygdala: from normal emotion to pathological anxiety. Behav Brain Res. 2011;223(2):403–10. doi: 10.1016/j.bbr.2011.04.025.

[61] Roy M, Shohamy D, Wager TD. Ventromedial prefrontal-subcortical systems and the generation of affective meaning. Trends Cogn Sci. 2012;16(3):147–56. doi: 10.1016/j.tics.2012.01.005.

[62] Klemm WR. Habenular and interpeduncularis nuclei: shared components in multiple-function networks. Med Sci Monit. 2004;10(11):RA261–73. http://www.MedSciMonit.com/pub/vol_10/no_11/4775.pdf.

[63] Viswanath H, Carter AQ, Baldwin PR, Molfese DL, Salas R. The medial habenula: still neglected. Front Hum Neurosci. 2014;7:931. doi: 10.3389/fnhum.2013.00931.

[64] Bianco IH, Wilson SW. The habenular nuclei: a conserved asymmetric relay station in the vertebrate brain. Philos Trans R Soc Lond B Biol Sci. 2009;364(1519):1005–20. doi: 10.1098/rstb.2008.0213.

[65] Sutherland RJ. The dorsal diencephalic conduction system: a review of the anatomy and functions of the habenular complex. Neurosci Biobehav Rev. 1982;6(1):1–13. doi: 10.1016/0149-7634(82)90003-3.

[66] Morley BJ. The interpeduncular nucleus. Int Rev Neurobiol. 1986;28:157–82.

[67] Bruinsma F, Loonen A. Neurobiology of cognitive and emotional motivation. Neuropraxis. 2006;10(3):77–88. doi: 10.1007/BF03079087.

[68] Heimer L. A new anatomical framework for neuropsychiatric disorders and drug abuse. Am J Psychiatry. 2003;160(10):1726–39. doi: 10.1176/appi.ajp.160.10.1726.

[69] Loonen AJ, Ivanova SA. New insights into the mechanism of drug-induced dyskinesia. CNS Spectr. 2013;18(1):15–20. doi: 10.1017/S1092852912000752.

[70] Groenewegen HJ. The basal ganglia and motor control. Neural Plast. 2003;10(1–2):107–20. doi: 10.1155/NP.2003.107.

[71] Groenewegen HJ, Trimble M. The ventral striatum as an interface between the limbic and motor systems. CNS Spectr. 2007;12(12):887–92. doi: 10.1017/S1092852900015650.

[72] Fuster JM. The prefrontal cortex. Fourth edition. Amsterdam: Academic Press, 2008.

[73] Stuss DT, Knight RT, eds. Principles of frontal lobe function. Oxford: Oxford University Press, 2002.

[74] Zald DH, Rauch SL, eds. The orbitofrontal cortex. Oxford: Oxford University Press, 2006.

[75] Rolls ET. The brain and emotion. Oxford, UK: University Press, 1999.

[76] Dalley JW, Mar AC, Economidou D, Robbins TW. Neurobehavioral mechanisms of impulsivity: fronto-striatal systems and functional neurochemistry. Pharmacol Biochem Behav. 2008;90(2):250–60. doi: 10.1016/j.pbb.2007.12.021.

[77] Loonen AJM, Stahl SM. The mechanism of drug-induced akathisia. CNS Spectr. 2011;16(1):7–10. doi: 10.1017/S1092852912000107.

[78] Nagai M, Kishi K, Kato S. Insular cortex and neuropsychiatric disorders: a review of recent literature. Eur Psychiatry. 2007;22(6):387–94. doi: 10.1016/j.eurpsy.2007.02.006.

[79] Hikosaka O. The habenula: from stress evasion to value-based decision-making. Nat Rev Neurosci. 2010;11(7):503–13. doi: 10.1038/nrn2866.

[80] Shabel SJ, Proulx CD, Trias A, Murphy RT, Malinow R. Input to the lateral habenula from the basal ganglia is excitatory, aversive, and suppressed by serotonin. Neuron. 2012;74(3):475–81. doi: 10.1016/j.neuron.2012.02.037.

[81] Poller WC, Madai VI, Bernard R, Laube G, Veh RW. A glutamatergic projection from the lateral hypothalamus targets VTA-projecting neurons in the lateral habenula of the rat. Brain Res. 2013;1507:45–60. doi: 10.1016/j.brainres.2013.01.029.

[82] Meye FJ, Lecca S, Valentinova K, Mameli M. Synaptic and cellular profile of neurons in the lateral habenula. Front Hum Neurosci. 2013;7:860. doi: 10.3389/fnhum.2013.00860.

[83] Kim U, Chang SY. Dendritic morphology, local circuitry, and intrinsic electrophysiology of neurons in the rat medial and lateral habenular nuclei of the epithalamus. J Comp Neurol. 2005;483(2):236–50. doi: 10.1002/cne.20410.

[84] Poletti M, Sambataro F. The development of delusion revisited: a transdiagnostic framework. Psychiatry Res. 2013;210(3):1245–59. doi: 10.1016/j.psychres.2013.07.032.

[85] Kapur S. Psychosis as a state of aberrant salience: a framework linking biology, phenomenology, and pharmacology in schizophrenia. Am J Psychiatry. 2003;160(1):13–23. doi: 10.1176/appi.ajp.160.1.13.

[86] Kapur S, Mizrahi R, Li M. From dopamine to salience to psychosis--linking biology, pharmacology and phenomenology of psychosis. Schizophr Res. 2005;79(1):59–68. doi: 10.1016/j.schres.2005.01.003.86.

[87] Kapur S, Agid O, Mizrahi R, Li M. How antipsychotics work-from receptors to reality. NeuroRx. 2006;3(1):10–21. doi: 10.1016/j.nurx.2005.12.003.

[88] Howes OD, Kapur S. The dopamine hypothesis of schizophrenia: version III--the final common pathway. Schizophr Bull. 2009;35(3):549–62. doi: 10.1093/schbul/sbp006.

[89] McGrath JJ, Saha S, Al-Hamzawi A, Alonso J, Bromet EJ, Bruffaerts R, Caldas-de-Almeida JM, Chiu WT, de Jonge P, Fayyad J, Florescu S, Gureje O, Haro JM, Hu C, Kovess-Masfety V, Lepine JP, Lim CC, Mora ME, Navarro-Mateu F, Ochoa S, Sampson N, Scott K, Viana MC, Kessler RC. Psychotic experiences in the general population: a cross-national analysis based on 31,261 respondents from 18 countries. JAMA Psychiatry. 2015;72(7):697–705. doi: 10.1001/jamapsychiatry.2015.0575.

[90] Kingston C, Schuurmans-Stekhoven J. Life hassles and delusional ideation: scoping the potential role of cognitive and affective mediators. Psychol Psychother. 2016. doi: 10.1111/papt.12089. [Epub ahead of print]

[91] van Os J. A salience dysregulation syndrome. Br J Psychiatry. 2009;194(2):101–3. doi: 10.1192/bjp.bp.108.054254.

[92] van Os J. 'Salience syndrome' replaces 'schizophrenia' in DSM-V and ICD-11: psychiatry's evidence-based entry into the 21st century?. Acta Psychiatr Scand. 2009;120(5):363–72. doi: 10.1111/j.1600-0447.2009.01456.x.

[93] van Os J. Are psychiatric diagnoses of psychosis scientific and useful? The case of schizophrenia. J Ment Health. 2010;19(4):305–17. doi: 10.3109/09638237.2010.492417.

[94] Loonen AJM. Mechanism of antipsychotic action - specific role of 5-HT2 and NMDA receptors. Tomsk, Novosibirsk, Barnaul, RU, 2014. www.researchgate.net doi: 10.13140/RG.2.1.2744.2323.

Chapter 7

Transcranial Magnetic Stimulation in Schizophrenia

Libor Ustohal, Tomas Sverak, Lenka Albrechtova,
Marie Hojgrova, Veronika Hublova and
Tomas Kasparek

Additional information is available at the end of the chapter

http://dx.doi.org/10.5772/65631

Abstract

Transcranial magnetic stimulation (TMS) is a method that can be used in neurophysiological research of schizophrenia and in the treatment of some symptoms or syndromes of this mental disorder. The most important indications for TMS (or repetitive TMS—rTMS) are the negative symptoms of schizophrenia and auditory hallucinations. Other less proven indications include cognitive deficit, especially working memory. This text summarizes general knowledge about (r)TMS and its use in schizophrenia. According to recent experiences, TMS is a very promising experimental and therapeutic method, but it needs further research for its optimized use.

Keywords: transcranial magnetic stimulation, TMS, rTMS, schizophrenia, negative symptoms, auditory hallucinations

1. Introduction

Transcranial magnetic stimulation (TMS) represents a relatively new method used in neurophysiological research, in which it helps to measure various cortical phenomena, including cortical inhibition, facilitation, and neuroplasticity. It is also used in the diagnosis and treatment of certain neuropsychiatric disorders. This method is a neurostimulation (neuromodulation) technique as is electroconvulsive therapy, vagal nerve stimulation, deep brain stimulation, transcranial direct current stimulation, and magnetic seizure therapy. Some neurostimulation techniques are invasive or semi-invasive; others, including TMS, are noninvasive [1, 2].

2. TMS principles, parameters and mechanism of action

The principle of the TMS method is based on Faraday's law of electromagnetic induction, formulated in 1831. This law states that around the primary coil through which a time-varying current is flowing, a changing magnetic field is created that is able to induce a secondary current in conductors found within its reach. A patient's brain may be one such conductor. The secondary current induced is, according to Lenz's law, in the direction opposing the primary current. During TMS, an insulated metal coil is placed over the patient's head that delivers a changing electrical current producing a changing magnetic field perpendicular to the current passing through the coil. Magnetic pulses may be administered individually (single-pulse TMS), or in pairs a few milliseconds apart (paired-pulse TMS), or repeatedly in a sequence or "train" lasting from seconds to minutes (repetitive transcranial magnetic stimulation or rTMS). The first two options are used primarily for research and diagnostic purposes; rTMS is used mainly in the treatment of certain neuropsychiatric disorders, including schizophrenia [1, 3].

Repetitive transcranial magnetic stimulation is defined by the number of pulses per second or by frequency in Hertz (Hz). The frequency is categorized as "low-frequency" ("slow") rTMS with 1 Hz or less and "high-frequency" ("fast") rTMS with more than 1 Hz (usually between 5 and 25 Hz). Another parameter of stimulation is its intensity expressed as the percentage of the individual resting motor threshold (MT). The motor threshold is defined as the minimal intensity of the stimulus able to produce muscle contraction in at least 5 of 10 successive trials (usually in one of the small muscles of the hand, e.g., the abductor pollicis brevis) when the stimulation is applied to the motor cortex. The most commonly used stimulation intensity varies between 80% and 120% of the individual resting motor threshold. Other stimulation parameters include the length of the train of pulses, the duration of the pause between them ("intertrain"), the total number of pulses administered during one session, the total number of individual sessions, the stimulation coil localization, the type of coil (the most commonly used type in rTMS is the "figure-of-eight coil"; there are also oval coils, conical coils etc.; the double cone coil is one of the most innovative types), and the coil's position, and orientation on the patient's head. The most frequent stimulation site is the dorsolateral prefrontal cortex (DLPFC). This stimulation site is usually defined as the location 5 cm rostral to the area of the motor cortex, the stimulation of which determines the resting motor threshold. Another method for the localization of the stimulation site uses the international system of EEG electrode placement 10/20; the most precise localization method is performed by stereotactic neuronavigation. An interesting modification of standard rTMS is pattern stimulation, with theta burst stimulation (TBS) as the most important [1–3].

Although the specific effect of rTMS on neurotransmission is not entirely clear, it has been proven repeatedly that high-frequency rTMS (10 to 20 Hz) increases brain excitability, and low-frequency rTMS (1 Hz and lower) decreases it. It has also been found that high-frequency rTMS applied over the left prefrontal cortex (PFC) increases brain perfusion, and thus the metabolism of this region, whereas low-frequency rTMS has the opposite effect [4].

http://dx.doi.org/10.5772/65631

3. TMS in neurophysiological research of schizophrenia

TMS with various single-pulse protocols and paired-pulse protocols is a useful tool for the assessment of physiology of the human motor system, including cortical excitability, inhibitory and excitatory mechanisms, conduction time, connectivity, and plasticity [5]. Moreover, Camprodon and Pascual-Leone [5] suppose that this tool has properties that we now need to understand across affective, behavioral, and cognitive circuits, to establish solid circuit-based models of neuropsychiatric diseases with the potential to affect clinical practice.

One of the phenomena, studied with TMS, is cortical inhibition. Cortical inhibition (CI) can be defined as a neurophysiological mechanism by which GABAergic interneurons influence the activity of other neurons. Several studies have identified CI impairment in schizophrenia. CI and CI impairment can be measured with a number of markers and protocols, including the cortical silent period (CSP). CSP measurement consists of a suprathreshold TMS pulse over the motor cortex paired with voluntary electromyographic activity, causing a cessation of muscle movement. The duration of this movement cessation is a measure of CI. It is thought that CSP measures $GABA_B$ inhibitory activity. Another CI marker is short-interval cortical inhibition (SICI). SICI measurement consists of a subthreshold conditioning TMS pulse preceding a suprathreshold pulse by several ms (1–5 ms). The amplitude of the motor-evoked potential (MEP) is then measured; it should be reduced by 50–90%. This marker is thought to measure $GABA_A$-mediated cortical inhibition [6–13]. Recent studies show that CI impairment can be improved with antipsychotics, especially clozapine, but also with quetiapine and risperidone [13–15]. Kaster et al. [13] suggested that the potentiation of $GABA_B$ may be a novel neurotransmitter mechanism that is involved in the pathophysiology and the treatment of schizophrenia. Another recent study found inhibitory deficits directly in the prefrontal cortex specific for schizophrenia using a combination of TMS and electroencephalography (EEG) [9]. Camprodon and Pascual-Leone [5] suppose that this multimodal combination of TMS and neuroimaging methods (EEG, magnetic resonance imaging, or positron emission tomography) can achieve TMS full potential—to measure the neurobiological effects of TMS even beyond the motor cortex.

4. Clinical application of TMS in schizophrenia

The most important use of TMS (or rTMS) is in the treatment of specific symptoms or syndromes of schizophrenia, especially negative symptoms and auditory hallucinations. Other less proven indications in schizophrenia include cognitive deficit, catatonic symptoms, obsessive-compulsive symptoms, and comorbid nicotine abuse (through the decrease of craving).

4.1. Negative symptoms

There is a consensus that the negative symptoms of schizophrenia include symptoms of affective flattening, alogia, avolition, social withdrawal, and anhedonia. The symptoms of inattention, poverty of content of speech, and inappropriate affect are also often assigned in measuring scales mainly due to the clinical evaluation of the overall disorganization seen in patients with schizophrenia [16].

Severity of negative symptoms in schizophrenia is usually linked with worse functional outcomes, including specific relationships with impaired occupational functioning, household integration, social functioning, engagement in recreational activities, and quality of life [16—18].

Negative symptoms are often associated with hypofrontality and with a lack of dopamine in the prefrontal cortex [19, 20].

4.1.1. Effect of rTMS in the prefrontal cortex

Some authors have found that high-frequency rTMS could increase cortical excitability and the metabolic activity of targeted neurons [21, 22]. Prefrontal rTMS also modulates dopamine release in the dorsal striatum and in the nucleus accumbens in Wistar rats [23]. High-frequency rTMS of the DLPFC induces the release of dopamine in the ipsilateral nucleus caudatus in healthy volunteers, and it causes downregulation of the 5-HT2 receptors in the frontal cortex [24, 25].

The change of the expression of glutamic acid decarboxylase, which is the synthetic enzyme of the precursor of GABA, could be also modified by rTMS. This finding may be important because the severity of negative symptoms has been found to be inversely related to benzodiazepine receptor binding in the medial frontal region [26].

These findings have led to the hypothesis that high-frequency rTMS applied at the prefrontal cortex may be an effective treatment of negative symptoms in schizophrenia, and many studies were published on this topic.

4.1.2. Current results of rTMS in the treatment of negative symptoms

We summarize in this text the results from three meta-analyses and from recent articles that are not a part of the last meta-analysis by Shi et al. [27].

The first meta-analysis reviewed eight double-blind studies and found that rTMS had a mild to moderate ($d = 0.58$) effect on alleviating the negative symptoms of schizophrenia [28]. The second meta-analysis evaluated nine double-blind studies with more than 200 enrolled patients [29]. When studies with any high-frequency stimulation of the left PFC were evaluated, the effect size of the treatment was low ($d = 0.43$); when the analysis included only studies with a 10 Hz frequency, the effect size of the treatment was intermediate ($d = 0.63$) [29]. The results of the third, most recent, meta-analysis suggest that rTMS is an effective treatment option for negative symptoms in schizophrenia. This meta-analysis included 16 studies. The moderators of rTMS on negative symptoms included duration of illness, stimulation frequency, stimulation intensity, and the type of outcome measures used (the effect size of rTMS on negative symptoms in sham-controlled trials was 0.80 as measured by the Scale for the Assessment of Negative Symptoms—SANS and 0.41 as measured by the Positive and Negative Syndrome Scale—PANSS) [27].

The authors of the third meta-analysis formulated some recommendations for the treatment of negative symptoms by rTMS based on the available results, which show that long-term stimulation (3 weeks or more) has a better effect than short-term stimulation. The best effect was with 10 Hz rTMS and 110% of individual MT. The number of pulses is also important—the effect is greater when the patient receives a higher number of pulses [27].

A recent study by Wobrock et al. included a sufficiently large sample (175 patients), but no statistically significant effect of rTMS was found in the improvement of negative symptoms in the active group compared with the sham group. The stimulation protocol was 15 sessions of 10 Hz stimulation of the left DLPFC, 110% MT, 5 s train and 30 s intertrain, and 15,000 pulses in the whole study. However, less-precise method was used for targeting the left DLPFC (the international system of EEG electrode placement 10/20, F3 electrode), and patients received a relatively small number of pulses, although the last meta-analysis indicated that a higher number of pulses have a better effect [30].

In another double-blind study, 117 patients with negative symptoms were randomized to a 20-day course of either active rTMS applied to the left DLPFC (it was targeted to 5 cm anterior to the point where maximum stimulation of the abductor pollicis brevis muscle was observed) or sham rTMS. The stimulation protocol was 10 Hz frequency, 4 s train and 56 s intertrain, 20 min each day, 80% MT, and 800 pulses per day. They reported that treatment with high-frequency rTMS for 6 weeks significantly improved negative symptoms in the active stimulation group as compared to the sham group. The decrease in negative symptoms persisted to the 6-month follow-up assessment [31].

Dlabac-de Lange et al. evaluated the effect of bilateral rTMS of DLPFC in schizophrenia patients with negative symptoms. The Tower of London (ToL) task during fMRI was used to measure the brain function of the DLPFC. The stimulation protocol was 10 Hz frequency, 15 sessions (divided into 3 weeks), 10 s train and 50 s intertrain, and 90% MT. Patients received 20 trains in one stimulation session. The brain activity in the right DLPFC and in the right medial frontal gyrus showed an increase in the active stimulation group after the stimulation, and the left posterior cingulate showed a decrease in brain activity after rTMS treatment of the DLPFC. No significant differences were found in task performance between the sham group and the active group after the treatment with rTMS. A significant difference was found in SANS but not in PANSS. The limits of the study can be seen in the localization of the DLPFC (targeted by F3 and F4 location from the EEG 10/20 system), in the small sample size (total of 24 patients) and in its heterogeneity, as there were significant differences between the active and sham groups at the beginning of the study [32].

4.1.3. New paradigms of rTMS in the treatment of negative symptoms

The authors of a recent study compared 96 patients who received 10 and 20 Hz, theta burst stimulation (TBS) and sham stimulation. The 10 Hz stimulation was only 80% MT at the beginning, and the intensity was gradually increased to 110% MT. Patients received 30 trains in one stimulation day, one stimulation interval was 5 s of the train and 30 s of the intertrain. The stimulation was divided into four weeks (20 stimulation sessions). The 20 Hz stimulation had the same stimulation parameters as the 10 Hz stimulation. In TBS, the basic train had a frequency of 5 Hz, and the stimulation was given every 200 ms. Three single pulses (50 Hz) were embedded within each 5 Hz pulse, on 80% MT, and each session had 2400 pulses. The TBS group had significantly larger reductions in SANS and PANSS negative subscale scores than the 10 Hz group and the 20 Hz group, but there were no significant differences in the two scales between the 10 and 20 Hz groups. There was a reduction in the scores in the mentioned scales in all groups with active stimulation compared with the sham group stimulation [33].

The cerebellum and cortico-thalamic-cerebellar circuit have also been included in the pathophysiology of schizophrenia. In patients with schizophrenia, some cerebellar dysfunctions were found, such as neurological soft signs, impaired eyeblink conditioning, procedural learning deficits, dyscoordination, abnormal posture, and poor cognitive performance. Resting state gamma activity is supposed to be a biomarker related to functional brain connectivity. One study tried to investigate the effect of cerebellar rTMS on resting state gamma activity. The efficacy of cerebellar rTMS was tested in 11 recent-onset schizophrenia patients who received 10 sessions of high-frequency rTMS to the midline cerebellum over a 2-week period. A significant decrease in negative symptoms and depression scores was observed after the rTMS treatment. Gamma spectral power in left frontal and temporal segments was reduced significantly after this treatment. In light of these preliminary results, cerebellar rTMS could be a useful innovation for the treatment of negative and affective symptoms in schizophrenia, but this has to be confirmed in further studies [34].

4.1.4. Negative symptoms and rTMS—summary

Recent guidelines state that high-frequency rTMS of the left DLPFC has a probable effect in the treatment of negative symptoms of schizophrenia (Level B evidence) [35].

A number of double-blind studies also proved a statistically significant decrease in the intensity of negative schizophrenia symptoms when current antipsychotic treatment was augmented with rTMS; the actual clinical significance of this procedure is disputed [4].

Another issue is represented by antipsychotic and other medication used in the treatment of patients with schizophrenia. According to some studies, this medication could negatively influence the activation induced by rTMS [36, 37].

rTMS represents a promising direction in the treatment of negative symptoms in schizophrenia, but it is necessary to improve current stimulation protocols (to use different frequencies in different areas, to investigate the effects of intensive stimulation protocols, and to investigate new targets such as the cerebellum).

4.2. Auditory hallucinations

Auditory verbal hallucinations (AVH), perceptions of voices in the absence of external stimuli, are a fundamental feature of mental illness and one of the characteristic symptoms of schizophrenia with high clinical importance [38]. AVH are reported by 50–70% of patients with schizophrenia, and in about 25–30% of patients, AVH are resistant to antipsychotic medication [39]. rTMS could be an additional therapeutic tool for AVH in schizophrenia [40].

4.2.1. *Effect of rTMS on auditory hallucinations*

The positive impact of rTMS on AVH can be seen in the inhibition of increased activity in the left temporoparietal cortex (TPC) (Broadmann area 40). This increased activity is repeatedly proven during hallucinations using brain imaging methods. This area is supposed to be involved in the perception of speech. The repeated stimulation of this area with a frequency of 1 Hz (low-frequency rTMS) induces a long-lasting decrease in the frequency and severity of medication-resistant AVH [41].

4.2.2. *Current results of clinical studies and meta-analyses*

The first study that applied rTMS as a therapeutic instrument for AVH was performed by Hoffman et al. in 1999. They postulated that low-frequency rTMS (1 Hz frequency) delivered to the left TPC would curtail auditory hallucinations by reducing the excitability of distributed neurocircuitry [39]. Since then several studies have been performed; some studies with positive results and others with negative results. All these studies were included in several meta-analyses.

The authors of the first meta-analysis observed a significant mean weighted effect size for rTMS versus sham stimulation, across 10 studies involving 212 patients ($d = 0.76$). The main outcome measure was the reduction in hallucinations as measured with appropriate psychometric rating scales. A typical hallucination rating scale is the Auditory Hallucinations Rating Scale (AHRS), which is a seven-item scale measuring frequency, reality, perceived loudness, number of different speaking voices, length of hallucinations (single words, phrases, sentences, or extended discourse), attentional salience (the degree to which hallucinations captured the attention of the patient), and distress level. When studies reported on multiple brain areas that were targeted with rTMS, only the left TPC was included. When only studies were included that used continuous stimulation (nine studies), the mean effect size increased to $d = 0.88$. To investigate whether the number of stimulation session would be an important variable, they compared studies with fewer than five stimulation sessions (four studies) to those with more than five stimulation sessions (six studies); there was no significant improvement. Two studies that included PANSS reported that rTMS had no significant effect on the PANSS positive subscale. Thus, the observed effect was specific to auditory hallucinations. There was no significant effect of rTMS on a composite index of general psychotic symptoms. The results provide support for the efficacy of the treatment in reducing the severity of AVH [42].

The second meta-analysis included ten studies with 232 patients. All these studies used low-frequency rTMS of the left TPC on patients with schizophrenia and treated and measured medication-resistant AVH. They extracted outcomes from several scales for assessing AVH: Hallucination Change Scale (HCS), Auditory Hallucinations Rating Scale (AHRS), Severity of Auditory Hallucinations (SAH scale), Psychotic Symptom Rating scale—Auditory Hallucinations Subscale (PSYRATS-AH), and Positive and Negative Syndrome Scale—Auditory Hallucinations Item (PANSS-AH). The HCS seems more sensitive to rTMS effects on AVH, while most studies using AHRS reported negative results. The authors observed significant effect size (Hedges' $g = 0.514$) [43].

The third meta-analysis was performed by Freitas et al. [28]. The authors specifically analyzed the effect on auditory hallucinations in seven sham-controlled studies and found a large and significant effect size for the sham-controlled studies (1.04; $p = 0.002$). They observed the need for individual assessment of the functional anatomy of hallucinations, using hallucination-activation maps obtained either by PET or fMRI, and stereotaxically determined the stimulation site following individual fMRI detection of inner speech regions instead of less sophisticated approach including coil position using the international 10/20 EEG electrode system in TP3 site, which might enhance TMS efficacy [43]. A critical finding in a study by Hoffman et al. concerned the discrepancy between the fMRI-guided TPC sites used in their trial and the standard TP3 which had little to no overlap [44]. Moreover, in a study by Sommer et al., five of the seven patients undergoing functional guided rTMS had predominant right-sided hallucinatory activity and were therefore stimulated over the right TPC [28, 45].

Another three meta-analyses were published by Slotema et al. [41, 46, 47]. According to the first one, with seven randomized controlled trials and 189 patients included, rTMS was superior to sham treatment, with a mean weighted effect size of 0.54 [46]. The second meta-analysis included 17 studies. The mean weighted effect size of rTMS directed at the left temporoparietal area was 0.44. But the effect of rTMS was no longer significant at one month of follow-up care (according to five studies with a follow-up assessment of at least one month) [47]. The most recent meta-analysis by Slotema included 19 studies with a total number of 548 patients. The mean weighted effect size for the treatment of auditory hallucinations was 0.44. No significant mean weighted effect size was found for the severity of psychosis. For patients with medication-resistant auditory hallucinations, the mean weighted effect size was 0.45. Repetitive transcranial magnetic stimulation applied at the left temporo-parietal area with a frequency of 1 Hz yielded a moderate mean weighted effect size of 0.63, indicating the superiority of this paradigm. Various other paradigms failed to show superior effects. rTMS applied at the right temporo-parietal area was not superior to sham treatment. The authors concluded that rTMS, especially when applied at the left temporo-parietal area with a frequency of 1 Hz, is effective for the treatment of auditory hallucinations, including for patients with medication-resistant hallucinations [41]. The limitation of all rTMS studies is the placebo, because of the difficulty of reproducing the noise and the scalp sensation (including superficial muscle contractions) of the active treatment. The initial method of producing a placebo effect was to tilt the coil at 45° or 90°. However, this method clearly unmasks it to patients who were previously treated with rTMS or for those in a crossover design. The more recent methods involve using a completely similar sham coil. Another significant limitation of these studies is the concomitant pharmacotherapy in all subjects. Several pharmacological treatments may interfere with treatment response, by modifying cortical excitability, by preventing the transsynaptic transmission of rTMS, or by interfering with the cerebral plasticity effects induced by rTMS [43].

4.2.3. Auditory hallucinations and rTMS—summary

The results of all of these meta-analyses show that 1 Hz rTMS applied at the left temporo-parietal area is effective in the treatment of auditory hallucinations (even in treatment-resistant patients), but the effect is of a relatively short duration (shorter than in patients with depressive disorder). In the trials covered in the meta-analysis by Slotema et al. [47], the effect of rTMS on AVH was no longer significant at the one-month follow-up visit. This short duration of the effect of rTMS is a matter of concern. A daily treatment of 2–4 weeks with a small treatment effect combined with a short duration may call into question its utility as a meaningful treatment for patients troubled by persistent symptoms [47]. The treatment of other positive symptoms with rTMS is ineffective. Recent guidelines state that low-frequency rTMS of the left TPC has a possible effect in the treatment of auditory hallucinations (Level C evidence); for other paradigms (high-frequency rTMS or continuous theta burst stimulation—cTBS), there are no recommendations [35].

4.3. Other indications

The treatment of other symptoms, syndromes, and comorbid conditions in patients with schizophrenia is less proven. Some studies focused on the cognitive effects of rTMS in schizophrenia. Their results were heterogeneous. A meta-analysis included four studies of high-frequency rTMS at the DLPFC and its effect on working memory. The authors concluded that rTMS significantly improved all measures of working memory performance [48]. But a recent study failed to prove a superior effect of rTMS over sham stimulation in the improvement of various cognitive domains in 156 schizophrenia patients with predominant negative symptoms [49]. Recent guidelines state no recommendations for the treatment of cognitive deficit in schizophrenia [35].

Three case studies described rTMS in the treatment of catatonic symptoms in patients with schizophrenia—the improvement in two cases was rapid and sufficient; the last case was negative [50].

A similar situation was seen in the treatment of obsessive-compulsive symptoms associated with schizophrenia. Two case studies with positive results were published, but the effect was only transient, and a recent pilot study had negative results [51, 52].

TMS offers an interesting option for the treatment of comorbid misuse of alcohol, nicotine, and other psychotropic substances. Two studies proved the effect of high-frequency rTMS at the left DLPFC on the reduction in cigarette consumption in patients with schizophrenia [53, 54].

TMS could also influence other less specific symptoms which are presents in schizophrenia as well as in other mental disorders, such as attention deficit or impulsiveness.

5. Future directions

It is possible to distinguish between two categories of factors associated with the efficacy of rTMS in schizophrenia: (1) clinical factors and (2) factors associated with rTMS, especially stimulation parameters.

Clinical factors include heterogeneity of symptoms of schizophrenia treated with rTMS, especially negative symptoms. Prikryl et al. analyzed negative symptoms influenced with rTMS using five domains of SANS (affective flattening/blunting, alogia, avolition/apathy, anhedonia, and impaired attention). The stimulation improved all domains, except for alogia [4]. To improve the results with rTMS, the definition and the prediction of responders are needed. This could be achieved using markers of impaired cortical inhibition and neuroplasticity—especially when TMS (with the potential to measure cortical inhibition and its changes) and EEG or other neuroimaging methods (MRI, fMRI, SPECT, PET) are combined. Tikka et al. described significant correlation between the reduction in negative and depressive symptoms in patients with schizophrenia and the reduction in gamma spectral power in left frontal and temporal segments after cerebellar rTMS. The authors suggest resting state gamma spectral power in frontal and temporal regions for a biomarker of treatment response [55]. Homan et al. described that responders were robustly differentiated from nonresponders to rTMS by the higher regional blood flow in the left superior temporal gyrus before treatment for AVH. The authors conclude that resting perfusion measurement before treatment might be a clinically relevant way to identify possible responders and nonresponders to rTMS [56].

The optimization of stimulation parameters is another important issue. New stimulation targets (for example, the cerebellum or anterior cingulate), better and more precise methods of stimulation coil placement (stereotactic navigation), new coil types (double cone coil, maybe H-coils for deep TMS), stimulation frequency (individual frequency), intensity, number of pulses (higher number of pulses), and the number of stimulation sessions (intensive stimulation) are also subjects of current research. This research can provide data for new and innovative stimulation paradigms, which are needed for a more robust clinical effect of TMS in schizophrenia.

6. Conclusion

TMS is a very promising research and therapeutic method for patients with schizophrenia. It is a useful tool for researching cortical inhibition and neuroplasticity. The most important application of TMS (or rTMS) is in the treatment of some symptoms or syndromes, especially negative symptoms (high-frequency rTMS at the left DLPFC) and auditory hallucinations (low-frequency rTMS at the left TPC), and maybe even cognitive deficit. The results of clinical studies are promising, but further research is needed to optimize the treatment results.

Acknowledgements

This work was supported by research grants from the Grant Agency of the Ministry of Health of the Czech Republic (AZV) NV15–30062A and NV15–31063A and by the Ministry of Health of the Czech Republic—conceptual development of research organization (FNBr, 65269705). The authors like to thank Ms. Anne Johnson for proof-reading.

http://dx.doi.org/10.5772/65631

Author details

Libor Ustohal[1,2*], Tomas Sverak[1,2], Lenka Albrechtova[1], Marie Hojgrova[1], Veronika Hublova[1] and Tomas Kasparek[1,2]

*Address all correspondence to: ustohal.libor@fnbrno.cz

1 Department of Psychiatry, Masaryk University and University Hospital Brno, Brno, Czech Republic

2 Central European Institute of Technology (CEITEC MU), Masaryk University, Brno, Czech Republic

References

[1] Ustohal L, Přikryl R, Přikrylová Kučerová H, Češková E. Repetitive transcranial magnetic stimulation (rTMS) in the treatment of depressive disorder. Activitas Nervosa Superior Rediviva 2011;53(1):3–13.

[2] Ustohal L, Valková B. Biological treatment methods in psychiatry – other methods. In: Hosák L, Hrdlička M, Libiger J, editors. Psychiatry and pedopsychiatry. 1st ed. Prague: Karolinum; 2016, p. 392–400.

[3] Burt T, Lisanby H, Sackeim H. Neuropsychiatric applications of transcranial magnetic stimulation: a meta-analysis. International Journal of Neuropsychopharmacology 2002;5(1):73–103.

[4] Prikryl R, Ustohal L, Prikrylova Kucerova H, Kasparek T, Venclikova S, Mayerova M, Ceskova E. A detailed analysis of the effect of repetitive transcranial magnetic stimulation on negative symptoms of schizophrenia: a double-blind trial. Schizophrenia Research 2013;149(1–3):167–173.

[5] Camprodon JA, Pascual-Leone A. Multimodal applications of transcranial magnetic stimulation for circuit-based psychiatry. JAMA Psychiatry 2016;73(4):407–408.

[6] Daskalakis ZJ, Christensen BK, Fitzgerald PB, Moller B, Fountain SI, Chen R. Increased cortical inhibition in persons with schizophrenia treated with clozapine. Journal of Psychopharmacology 2008;22(2):203–209.

[7] Liu SK, Fitzgerald PB, Daigle M, Chen R, Daskalakis ZJ. The relationship between cortical inhibition, antipsychotic treatment, and the symptoms of schizophrenia. Biological Psychiatry 2009;65(6):503–509.

[8] Radhu N, de Jesus DR, Ravindran LN, Zanjani A, Fitzgerald PB, Daskalakis ZJ. A meta-analysis of cortical inhibition and excitability using transcranial magnetic stimulation in psychiatric disorders. Clinical Neurophysiology 2013;124:1309–1320.

[9] Radhu N, Garcia Dominguez L, Farzan F, Richter MA, Semeralul MO, Chen R, et al. Evidence for inhibitory deficits in the prefrontal cortex in schizophrenia. Brain 2015;138:483–497.

[10] Rogasch NC, Daskalakis ZJ, Fitzgerald PB. Cortical inhibition, excitation, and connectivity in schizophrenia: a review of insights from transcranial magnetic stimulation. Schizophrenia Bulletin 2014;40(3):685–696.

[11] Fuhr P, Agostino R, Hallett M. Spinal motor neuron excitability during the silent period after cortical stimulation. Electroencephalography and Clinical Neurophysiology 1991;81(4):257–262.

[12] Kujirai T, Caramia MD, Rothwell JC, Day BL, Thompson PD, Ferbert A, et al. Corticocortical inhibition in human motor cortex. Journal of Physiology 1993;471:501–519.

[13] Kaster TS, de Jesus D, Radhu N, Farzan F, Blumberger DM, Rajji TK, et al. Clozapine potentiation of GABA mediated cortical inhibition in treatment resistant schizophrenia. Schizophrenia Research 2015;165:157–162.

[14] Frank E, Landgrebe M, Poeppl TB, Schecklmann M, Kreuzer PM, Prasser J, et al. Antipsychotic treatment with quetiapine increases the cortical silent period. Schizophrenia Research 2014;156:128–132.

[15] Ustohal L, Mayerova M, Hublova V, Prikrylova Kucerova H, Ceskova E, Kasparek T. Risperidone increases the cortical silent period in drug-naive patients with first-episode schizophrenia: a transcranial magnetic stimulation study. Journal of Psychopharmacology 2016 Aug 15:1–5. pii: 0269881116662650. [Epub ahead of print]

[16] Foussias G, Agid O, Fervaha G, Remington G. Negative symptoms of schizophrenia: clinical features, relevance to real world functioning and specificity versus other CNS disorders. European Neuropsychopharmacology 2014;24(5):693–709.

[17] Hunter R, Barry S. Negative symptoms and psychosocial functioning in schizophrenia: neglected but important targets for treatment. European Psychiatry 2012;27(6):432–436.

[18] Leifker FR, Bowie CR, Harvey PD. Determinants of everyday outcomes in schizophrenia: the influences of cognitive impairment, functional capacity, and symptoms. Schizophrenia Research 2009;115(1):82–87.

[19] Gonul AS, Kula M, Eşel E, Tutuş A, Sofuoglu S. A Tc-99m HMPAO SPECT study of regional cerebral blood flow in drug-free schizophrenic patients with deficit and non-deficit syndrome. Psychiatry Research: Neuroimaging 2003;123(3):199–205.

[20] Hill K, Mann L, Laws KR, Stephenson CM, Nimmo-Smith I, McKenna PJ. Hypofrontality in schizophrenia: a meta-analysis of functional imaging studies. Acta Psychiatrica Scandinavica 2004;110(4):243–256.

[21] Eisenegger C, Treyer V, Fehr E, Knoch D. Time-course of "off-line" prefrontal rTMS effects—a PET study. NeuroImage 2008;42(1):379–384.

[22] Speer AM, Kimbrell TA, Wassermann EM, D Repella J, Willis MW, Herscovitch P, Post RM. Opposite effects of high and low frequency rTMS on regional brain activity in depressed patients. Biological Psychiatry 2000;48(12):1133–1141.

[23] Keck ME, Welt T, Müller MB, Erhardt A, Ohl F, Toschi N, et al. Repetitive transcranial magnetic stimulation increases the release of dopamine in the mesolimbic and mesostriatal system. Neuropharmacology 2002;43(1):101–109.

[24] Strafella AP, Paus T, Barrett J, Dagher A. Repetitive transcranial magnetic stimulation of the human prefrontal cortex induces dopamine release in the caudate nucleus. The Journal of Neuroscience: The Official Journal of the Society for Neuroscience 2001;21(15):RC157.

[25] Ben-Shachar D, Gazawi H, Riboyad-Levin J, Klein E. Chronic repetitive transcranial magnetic stimulation alters b-adrenergic and 5-HT2 receptor characteristics in rat brain. Brain Research 1999;816(1):78–83.

[26] Busatto GF, Pilowsky LS, Costa DC, Ell PJ, David AS, Lucey JV, Kerwin RW. Correlation between reduced in vivo benzodiazepine receptor binding and severity of psychotic symptoms in schizophrenia. American Journal of Psychiatry 1997;154(1):56–63.

[27] Shi C, Yu X, Cheung EFC, Shum DHK, Chan RCK. Revisiting the therapeutic effect of rTMS on negative symptoms in schizophrenia: a meta-analysis. Psychiatry Research 2013;215(3):505–513.

[28] Freitas C, Fregni F, Pascual-Leone A. Meta-analysis of the effects of repetitive transcranial magnetic stimulation (rTMS) on negative and positive symptoms in schizophrenia. Schizophrenia Research 2009;108(1–3):11–24.

[29] Dlabac-de Lange JJ, Knegtering R, Aleman A. Repetitive transcranial magnetic stimulation for negative symptoms of schizophrenia: review and meta-analysis. The Journal of Clinical Psychiatry 2010;71(4):411–418.

[30] Wobrock T, Guse B, Cordes J, Wölwer W, Winterer G, Gaebel W, et al. Left prefrontal high-frequency repetitive transcranial magnetic stimulation for the treatment of schizophrenia with predominant negative symptoms: a sham-controlled, randomized multicenter trial. Biological Psychiatry 2015;77(11):979–988.

[31] Quan WX, Zhu XL, Qiao H, Zhang WF, Tan SP, Zhou DF, Wang XQ. The effects of high-frequency repetitive transcranial magnetic stimulation (rTMS) on negative symptoms of schizophrenia and the follow-up study. Neuroscience Letters 2015;584: 197–201.

[32] Dlabac-de Lange JJ, Liemburg EJ, Bais L, Renken RJ, Knegtering H, Aleman A. Effect of rTMS on brain activation in schizophrenia with negative symptoms: a proof-of-principle study. Schizophrenia Research 2015;168(1–2):475–482.

[33] Zhao S, Kong J, Li S, Tong Z, Yang C, Zhong H. Randomized controlled trial of four protocols of repetitive transcranial magnetic stimulation for treating the negative symptoms of schizophrenia. Shanghai Archives of Psychiatry 2014;26(1):15–21.

[34] Sayar GH, Bulut H, Nevzat T. Use of repetitive transcranial magnetic stimulation in treatment of negative symptoms of schizophrenia. Journal of Neurology, Neurological Science and Disorders 2015;1(1):17–21.

[35] Lefaucheur J, André-Obadia N, Antal A, Ayache SS, Baeken C, Benninger DH, et al. Evidence-based guidelines on the therapeutic use of repetitive transcranial magnetic stimulation (rTMS). Clinical Neurophysiology 2014;125(11):2150–2206.

[36] Abbott C, Juárez M, White T, Gollub RL, Pearlson GD, Bustillo J, et al. Antipsychotic dose and diminished neural modulation: a multi-site fMRI study. Progress in Neuro-Psychopharmacology and Biological Psychiatry 2011;35(2):473–482.

[37] Hasan A, Falkai P, Wobrock T. Transcranial brain stimulation in schizophrenia: targeting cortical excitability, connectivity and plasticity. Current Medicinal Chemistry 2013;20(3):405–413.

[38] Dierks T, Linden DEJ, Jandl M, Formisano E, Goebel R, Lanfermann H, et al. Activation of Heschl's Gyrus during Auditory Hallucinations. Neuron 1999;22(3):615–621.

[39] Hoffman RE, Boutros NN, Hu S, Berman RM, Krystal JH, Charney DS. Transcranial magnetic stimulation and auditory hallucinations in schizophrenia. Lancet 2000;355(9209):1073–1075.

[40] de Weijer AD, Sommer IE, Lotte Meijering A, Bloemendaal M, Neggers SF, Daalman K, Boezeman EH. High frequency rTMS; a more effective treatment for auditory verbal hallucinations? Psychiatry Research 2014;224(3):204–210.

[41] Slotema CW, Blom JD, Van Lutterveld R, Hoek HW, Sommer IEC. Review of the efficacy of transcranial magnetic stimulation for auditory verbal hallucinations. Biological Psychiatry 2014;76(2):101–110.

[42] Aleman A, Sommer IE, Kahn RS. Efficacy of slow repetitive transcranial magnetic stimulation in the treatment of resistant auditory hallucinations in schizophrenia: a meta-analysis. Journal of Clinical Psychiatry 2007;68(3):416–421.

[43] Tranulis C, Sepehry AA, Galinowski A, Stip E. Should we treat auditory hallucinations with repetitive transcranial magnetic stimulation? A metaanalysis. Canadian Journal of Psychiatry. Revue Canadienne De Psychiatrie 2008;53(9):577–586.

[44] Hoffman RE, Hampson M, Wu K, Adam W, Gore JC, Buchanan RJ, et al. probing the pathophysiology of auditory/verbal hallucinations by combining functional magnetic

resonance imaging and transcranial magnetic stimulation. Cerebral Cortex 2007;17(11): 2733–2743.

[45] Sommer IEC, Slotema CW, de Weijer AD, Blom JD, Daalman K, Neggers SF, et al. Can fMRI-guidance improve the efficacy of rTMS treatment for auditory verbal hallucinations? Schizophrenia Research 2007;93(1–3):406–408.

[46] Slotema CW, Blom JD, Hoek HW, Sommer IEC. Should we expand the toolbox of psychiatric treatment methods to include Repetitive Transcranial Magnetic Stimulation (rTMS)? A meta-analysis of the efficacy of rTMS in psychiatric disorders. Journal of Clinical Psychiatry 2010;71(7):873–884.

[47] Slotema CW, Aleman A, Daskalakis ZJ, Sommer IE. Meta-analysis of repetitive transcranial magnetic stimulation in the treatment of auditory verbal hallucinations: update and effects after one month. Schizophrenia Research 2012;142(1–3):40–45.

[48] Brunoni AR, Vanderhasselt MA. Working memory improvement with non-invasive brain stimulation of the dorsolateral prefrontal cortex: a systematic review and meta-analysis. Brain and Cognition 2014;86:1–9.

[49] Hasan A, Guse B, Cordes J, Wölwer W, Winterer G, Gaebel W. Cognitive effects of high-frequency rTMS in schizophrenia patients with predominant negative symptoms: results from a multicenter randomized sham-controlled trial. Schizophrenia Bulletin 2016;42(3):608–618.

[50] Trojak B, Meille V, Bonin B, Chauvet-Geliner JC. Repetitive transcranial magnetic stimulation for the treatment of catatonia: an alternative treatment to electroconvulsive therapy? Journal of Neuropsychiatry and Clinical Neurosciences 2014;26(2):E42–E43.

[51] Mendes-Filho VA, Belmonte de Abreu P, Pedrini M, Cachoeira CT, Lobato MI. rTMS as an add-on treatment for resistant obsessive-compulsive symptoms in patients with schizophrenia: report of three cases. Revista Brasileira de Psiquiatria 2013;35(2):210–211.

[52] Mendes-Filho VA, de Jesus DR, Belmonte-de-Abreu P, Cachoeira CT, Rodrigues Lobato MI. Effects of repetitive transcranial magnetic stimulation over supplementary motor area in patients with schizophrenia with obsessive-compulsive-symptoms: a pilot study. Psychiatry Research 2016;242:34–38.

[53] Wing VC, Bacher I, Wu BS, Daskalakis ZJ, George TP. High frequency repetitive transcranial magnetic stimulation reduces tobacco craving in schizophrenia. Schizophrenia Research 2014;139(1–3):264–266.

[54] Prikryl R, Ustohal L, Kucerova HP, Kasparek T, Jarkovsky J, Hublova V, Vrzalova M, Ceskova E. Repetitive transcranial magnetic stimulation reduces cigarette consumption in schizophrenia patients. Progress in Neuro-Psychopharmacology and Biological Psychiatry 2014;49:30–35.

[55] Tikka SK, Garg S, Sinha VK, Nizamie SH, Goyal N. Resting state dense array gamma oscillatory activity as a response marker for cerebellar-repetitive transcranial magnetic stimulation (rTMS) in schizophrenia. Journal of ECT 2015;31(4):258–262.

[56] Homan P, Kindler J, Hauf M, Hubl D, Dierks T. Cerebral blood flow identifies responders to transcranial magnetic stimulation in auditory verbal hallucinations. Translational Psychiatry 2012;2:e189.

Chapter 8

Sport: A Possible Road toward Social Inclusion and Quality of Life

Maria Cristina Turola, Davide Barbieri,
Angelo Palazzi, Veronica Pallotta, Luciana Simani,
Chiara Tosi and Ombretta Zanardi

Additional information is available at the end of the chapter

http://dx.doi.org/10.5772/65632

Abstract

Sport is a universal language, recognized and shared by all. A psychiatric users Association, in collaboration with public Mental Health Department and UISP, Italian Union Promoting Sport for All, proposes the sport as one of the possible strategies within a wider therapeutic project for schizophrenia. Soft gymnastic, swimming, football, and volley are observed from the point of view of users, main recipients of the intervention, trainers, and referees. The perceived quality of life was measured in the users/athletes, using the WHOQOL-brief schedule. To practice sport enhances the adhesion to treatment and the quality of life and can reduce hospitalizations. It is a useful tool for promoting well-being, personal autonomy and an active lifestyle, preventing isolation, and improving self-esteem and social cognition. It may be an important factor preventing poor functional outcome and promoting recovery. Team sports seem to have a greater therapeutic value, producing fun, cohesion, and social inclusion; they can also play an important educational role, preventing social stigma.

Keywords: sport, schizophrenia, functional outcome, self-esteem, social cognition, quality of life, psychiatric users

1. Introduction

The schizophrenic disorders show a very diverse spectrum for symptoms, manifestations, abilities/disabilities both personal and in the different aspects of relational and social life, experiences and self-perceiving, and external points of view, including those of family members and practitioners, judgments, and prejudices of society.

The transition from a hospital care model, almost always based on seclusion, to a territorial care model has eliminated the artifacts of institutionalization, allowing to highlight the wide range of individual differences in the onset, course, and outcome of the disease. It is impossible to apply a unique model of approach and therapy; instead, it is essential to work using individual projects, which should be adapted to the evolution over time of the person-disease-care system. In Italy, the model of nonhospital psychiatric assistance is now being implemented by almost 40 years, allowing to accumulate an enormous asset of experiences and expertise in a system in which everyone plays an active role: patients, better defined as users, family members, practitioners and psychiatric workers, associations, schools, and other agencies of civil society.

The challenge of the last years is not the treatment of the symptoms, which, at least for the positive symptoms, finds a wide range of effective drugs: the challenge is to recreate or to build up *ex novo* personal skills and social relationships networks, to find a valuable role in society, and to achieve a satisfactory quality of life. To achieve these objectives is an ambitious, but possible, goal, and requires employing all the available resources. In this context, a psychiatric users Association proposes the sport as one of the possible strategies within a wider therapeutic project for schizophrenia. The main characteristic of this work is that schizophrenic disorders and sport as a method of rehabilitation and social inclusion are observed first of all from the point of view of users, main recipients of the intervention: subsequently, they have broadened the point of view, involving other figures that operate in this project: psychiatric workers, facilitators, trainers, referees, family members, teachers and students, local Authorities, and other associations.

2. Background and caseload

2.1. Population, Mental Health Department and schizophrenia

The province of Ferrara, in the Emilia-Romagna region (Italy), has a population of around 360,000 inhabitants. The treatment of psychiatric disorders is guaranteed by the Local Public Health Agency of Ferrara, through the Mental Health Department (MHD), using the community care model. The territory has an important feature in offering personalized care paths and on relies to hospitalization only in the case of onset of acute symptoms that cannot be treated as outpatients.

The treatment path uses different instruments: medical and nursing interviews, drug therapy, psychoeducational groups, cognitive groups, expressive therapies, family intervention, and proposals for enrolling in specific training programs stage.

People affected by schizophrenia spectrum disorders are diagnosed and taken over by the MHD Territorial Service, which starts a personalized treatment plan and carries it on over time,

http://dx.doi.org/10.5772/65632

referring also, where necessary, to rehabilitative semi-residential or residential programs or to short-term hospitalization (average 11 days) in acute pathology ward. In recent years, it was also initiated a very interesting departmental project of early intervention for psychosis [1].

In 2009–2010 [2], a systematic evaluation of all people affected by schizophrenia spectrum disorders [category 295 of International Classification of Diseases (ICD9)], in charge of the provincial MHD, allowed to get several important and useful information. The cases were 842: 486 males and 356 females, with an average observation time of 13 years.

The research considered both symptoms, evaluated using the Brief Psychiatric Rating Scale (BPRS) 24 item [3] and personal/social functioning evaluated using the Personal and Social Performance Scale (PSP) [4]. Only 5.3% of cases showed severe symptoms versus 78% of cases asymptomatic or mildly symptomatic. Conversely, the evaluation of personal and social functioning evidenced, in the sample, a widespread situation of disability, with relevant difficulties in one-half of cases in the work/social utility area and in personal relationships area. There were statistical significant gender differences with males less able than females.

A very important result of this research is that course and outcome of the disease are not affected by early onset or long disease duration: the possibility of improvement or healing exists for all cases, even those with a long history of illness and hospitalizations.

2.2. The psychiatric users association

Club Integriamoci NGO Association, based in Ferrara, was founded in 1998 by a group of psychiatric users and former users, psychiatric workers, and volunteers.

In the early years of the association, the psychiatric workers have provided a constant presence and played a very important role, supporting users in their path toward autonomy: they started activities, participated in them, and identified the most suitable users carrying out management functions or activities conductors. Many activities and projects were also financially supported by the MHD. Over the years, manual and craft activities have been carried out, especially for females and a 3-year theater project as part of a European project of which the town of Ferrara was partner.

Currently, the Association is completely managed by the users, who hold all the management positions, perform administrative functions, and take all decisions as a group and plan together the activities and initiatives. The main activity of the association has always been and nowadays is to practice sports, in collaboration with the Mental Health Department, the UISP (Italian Union Promoting Sport for All) and the Municipality of Ferrara. The Association participates in further outdoor activities, especially hiking, walking, and bike riding, as part of a regional project ("Moving Citizens 2") that promotes physical activity outdoors.

The Association undertakes activities of information and contrasting stigma, especially in high schools: testimonies, but also volleyball or football matches. Moreover, it participates in regional sport tournament and collaborates with different NGO Association in ethical projects.

3. Method

The Mental Health treating team performs the referral to the sport activity with different objectives as to promote health and physical well-being, to motivate social participation and prevent isolation, to have recurring weekly activity, and to socialize or to promote specific personal and relational skills or social integration.

The technical aspects of training are supervised by professional coaches provided by UISP, while the weekly organization and conduction of sports activities, initiated by psychiatric workers and conducted by them for over 10 years, are since 3 years assigned to a user with specific training as a social facilitator, who is always present. The facilitator is a user who has achieved a good level of clinical stabilization and who is perceived by other users as an ally, able to understand their feelings, because he too has had experiences. At the same time, he is the referee of fairness of play in the field and guarantees the respect of sporting rules; he acts as a mediator among the athletes and acts as a liaison between them and the MHD staff.

The psychiatric worker, belonging to the MHD semi-residential rehabilitation center, collaborates with the social facilitator for the implementation of sports activities and works together with the caring team when admitting the new users/athletes; she supervises and maintains links with MHD and regional sports groups. Facilitator and psychiatric worker together reinforce the results obtained with the sports, promote self-esteem, create the conditions allowing everyone to feel at ease and find a role in the activities. They closely cooperate in the organization and coordination of activities, as required by a specific protocol of collaboration.

Sports activities as part of a therapeutic rehabilitation project are currently four: at an individual level, gymnastics and swimming in the pool, and as a team, volleyball and football (5 or 11 players). To these activities take part weekly about 50 people, males and females, aged between 20 and 64 years, with different psychiatric disorders; schizophrenia represents more than half of the diagnoses. Many users/athletes practice currently more than one activity.

All sports are practiced at least once a week; in addition to this, we organize and take part to social events and regional sport meeting. At least once a month, the volleyball and soccer teams play against teams of high schools, as part of a project aiming to educate young people and fight stigma. Sport activities are subject to either external observation—by professional coaches, psychiatric worker and facilitator—and self-observation by athletes themselves. In team sports, the end of a session of training is often followed by a time of reflection, informal but very effective, where the team group examines the progress achieved and any difficulties encountered, and programs the next workout or the participation in tournaments.

To gather more information, the point of view of users athletes has been audited in 2016 with individual interviews and using the World Health Organization Quality of Life (WHOQOL)-brief schedule, 26 items [5], to get information about the perceived level of quality of life.

http://dx.doi.org/10.5772/65632

4. Sport

"Sports have the power to change the world. It has the power to inspire, the power to unite people in a way that little else does. It speaks to youth in a language they understand. Sports can create hope, where there was once only despair. It is more powerful than governments in breaking down racial barriers. It laughs in the face of all types of discrimination" said Nelson Mandela in 2000 [6].

Sport as an ideal value [7] was born in ancient Greece, where the Olympic Games were the occasion of peaceful encounter, and not confrontation, among people who recognized themselves in a common identity, while belonging to different political or social systems. During the games, conflicts were suspended, gift was exchanged, and all people had to follow common law, as the possibility of participation for all; misbehaviors were prevented or punished.

In contemporary culture, sport is a total cultural phenomenon that has transformed social customs and even the clothes; it involves everyday life context, it is magnified out of proportion by the media, and it reflects, at a different level, the same problems and contradictions of the society. It is no longer a value in itself; rather it is often a source of conflict, confrontation, and aggression.

It becomes a "value" only within an ethical and educational context, when it takes a positive social meaning and promotes the good of the community and the improvement of relations among its members [8]. The Recommendation on the European Sport for All Charter, adopted in 1992 and revised in 2001 [9] defines sport as a right for all citizens, of which the States must be guarantors; moreover, it recognizes "the diverse contributions which sport can make to personal and social development."

For people with disabilities, whether physical or mental, sports are not always easy: it is necessary to overcome resistance and personal or environmental barriers. Sometimes, one has to use devices, or even build them. Sometimes, it is necessary to adapt the rules, so that they may become accessible, to find the facilities but, above all, it is essential to find organizations available to welcome individual athletes or groups of athletes with disabilities and their needs. For isolated people this is very difficult; the presence of corporate associations, connected in a network of associations, increases the possibilities and sport opportunities.

In physical disability, injury or sensory loss is visible and obvious; in this area, sport is now universally recognized as a therapeutic, rehabilitative tool of socialization and inclusion. The high costs of devices are certainly an obstacle, but there is usually a strong motivation of the athletes, their family and social environment. Adapted Sport [10] plays an important role both at school and in leisure and free time, while the Paralympics events [11], with their large participation of athletes and public, are a powerful media instrument of sport values in conditions of disability.

In mental disability, impairment is not immediately visible, and devices are not necessary, but it is often necessary to adapt the rules of the different sports. In most cases, sports activities are carried out within the Psychiatric Services, for recreational and therapeutic purposes; for young people, there are special projects in schools, especially in high schools.

Networks of Associations promote sport at a regional level or national one: some Associations are strongly characterized in the health-psychiatric domain (i.e., ANPIS, Plural Sport Association for Social Integration); others operate in an "external" field the civil society. Among these, the UISP is the most common, but there are many others. Intellectual and Relational Disability Federation (FISDIR) is affiliated with the Paralympic Committee.

The concrete work in this area is extremely widespread, at least in Italy, with a wide range of popular sports: athletics, gymnastics, swimming, skiing, sailing, canoeing and rowing, archery, bocce, judo, tennis, table tennis, football, basketball, volleyball, and rugby. In our limited experience, we are aware of a dozen soccer teams and more than twenty volleyball teams, we have reports of various regional tournaments and even a regular UISP championship, in the Piemonte Region.

4.1. Our practiced sports

4.1.1. Soft gymnastics

Soft gymnastic was born in the seventies of the last century, as a set of activities aimed at finding a harmonious relationship with the body and the environment, through a conscious and active working attitude. It is a misleading to consider it as an application of traditional exercise in a reduced scale, for "weak" people.

Our body is very sensitive to anything that can alter its equilibrium. If one makes a pleasant experience and enjoys feelings of well-being, it will try to reproduce these feelings in an unconsciousness manner; on the contrary, bad experiences and unpleasant feelings will lead to painful muscle contractions and poor posture. Therefore, it is important to learn to feel and know every sensation coming from the body, to become aware of the movement, and to adopt personal strategies contrasting physical and psychological distress.

Anyone can enjoy soft gymnastics, regardless of age, even in non-homogeneous age groups; the perfect setting for these activities is a heated gym with a wooden or rubber silent floor, in order to favor listening and concentration. There is no need for special equipment, except for mats and small equipment, such as balls or tennis balls, which facilitate the work on the perception of the body.

Our gymnastics groups, attended by about thirty people, males and females, are held weekly and are led by a UISP teacher with special training. Each lesson lasts between 50 and 60 min and is divided into three sections: worm up, work, and cooldown. During worm up, we execute full body preparation exercises, aimed at further improvement of equilibrium, muscle tone, coordination, and proprioception. After the warm up, there is a phase in which participants stand in circle to be able to face each other. This produces a greater degree of harmony and the creation of a group in which all feel an integrative part.

Exercises and movements are taken from different techniques, all aiming to restore the psychophysical equilibrium and the harmony of the body: Eutonia, or Alexander method [12], Bertherat "anti-gymnastic"[13], Feldenkrais method [14], and Stretching.

The final phase, body relaxation, allows to reach a physical and psychological well-being. We also use music as a basis to facilitate individual expressiveness and build a body-mind feedback that generates positive reactions.

The teacher carries out both an individual and group observation, periodically evaluates eventual problems, improvements and acquisitions of skills, highlighting especially the qualitative aspects of the movement. Other objectives of soft exercise are to improve psychological well-being and ability to manage stress, to reduce anxiety, and to improve self-esteem and social integration. An important goal is also to create a positive and welcoming environment, encouraging the formation of a good group, and allowing to achieve harmony and well-being among all participants.

4.1.2. Swimming

In swimming, the main factor is water, with its physical characteristics (hydrostatic pressure, temperature, buoyancy) that interacts with the body. Our classes, involving 12 people, males and females, are conducted on a weekly basis in an indoor pool, 1.30 m deep, under the guidance of a professional UISP instructor. The sessions include a technical phase, in groups, related to different swimming styles (crawl, backstroke, breaststroke), and a phase of free swimming for those who have already acquired skills. Also diving activities are carried out in group, in a circle, and so is final relaxation, using schemes like the horse water or the fish star.

A preliminary difficulty, for some people, is made up of having to undress, and show a body that does not meet the prevailing standards of beauty, or a shape which is different from your "ideal" body, that of youth or before illness: leaner, more muscular, straighter, maybe more tanned. Some women have implemented an effective strategy to deal with this problem, wearing different costumes, such as those for diving.

To get in the pool is, for some people, an already known experience, mostly pleasant: they are good swimmers and they are happy to be in the water. For others, it's a new experience and it can also be scary for the loss of contact with the earth, for fear of sinking, for the difficulty of letting go to support of water, and for the loss of the usual boundaries.

Once entered in the water, the cutaneous perceptions change: most of the body surface is no longer surrounded from the air, but by a liquid, which exerts a pressure on the skin, and which has a temperature that may be important for the purposes of the first adaptation.

People must also deal with the effect of buoyancy on every single human body, depending on the shape, the weight and body density: some parts tend to float and others, with a greater relative weight, tend to sink. Flotation entails a different equilibrium, which will vary with the slightest movement, inducing continuous adaptations in the proprioceptive perception system. This changes completely the entire movement control and coordination, according to new parameters, not usual in a "dry" environment.

The decrease in the gravity for the effect of water leads to a feeling of lightness, which is generally pleasant. For the same reasons, this environment is particularly suitable for mobilization and a gradual cardio-respiratory training in people with weight problems, condition often associated with psychotic disorders, especially chronic.

Among the benefits of the activity in the pool, we note especially the possibility of enhance movement and coordination and the feeling of psychological well-being, helpful in decreasing anxiety. To attend a swimming pool, with its rules of use, helps to take a greater care of self. In addition, being able to carry out a complex activity and learn new skills improves self-esteem, while to take part of a group fosters communication.

4.1.3. Football and 5-players football

In our Association, currently, we have only male players: fifteen people with age ranging from 21 to 57 years (older people are goalkeepers). Football is a sport that readily attracts new young users, as known and socially widespread and appreciated. In the version with 11 players, it requires good physical condition and enough breath to run across the field, as well as a certain level of technical ability. Everyone seems to have previous experience; they all had play as children: on outdoor courts, at school or after the school.

In the 5-players version of the game, the field is much smaller, and the spaces are narrower, with more frequent contacts among the players; breathing capacity becomes less important, while control of the ball and quick overview of the field, teammates, and opponents becomes more important. The game is dynamic and fast, and there is the possibility of some injury due to the accidental knocks or falls; risks of accident are taken into account from the very beginning. The main problem of football is the physical contact between players, and its possible meaning—not openly declared—of aggressive behavior.

In our team, the starting rules, shared and accepted by all, are simple and clear: to play for fun and you can win or lose; it makes no sense to get angry with you or with teammates. Teams are not fixed, but they are decided from time to time. The instructor looks after the technical aspects, while the facilitator is the guarantor of fairness in the field. If the aggressiveness increase, the facilitator gives a first call; then, if the problem persists, he stops the game and sends all in the locker room.

The football team plays once a month against a representative of the Ferrara Scientific High School and participates in several tournaments in the area of Mental Health or during local events.

4.1.4. Volleyball

More than twenty people take part to Volley activity, males and females, aged from 27 to 60 years. This sport is easy to understand: at the basic level, people of all ages and fitness levels can participate, sometimes eventually using small adjustments, such as the stroke from inside the field.

Volley promotes correct behavior in the field and the respect of the opponent to the point that the team who protests or offends the referee loses the point. It has also the great advantage of keeping teams separate, each in own field, with a net between the two teams and the two halves of the field. The net allows to see the opposing team, but there is no body contact; only the ball can pass from one field to the other, always in the air, in flight; who let it drop loses the point.

The error is a normal occurrence in the course of the game: the team who makes fewer mistakes wins the match. It is an exquisitely collaborative game: all players bring a contribution. To know the playmates and their characteristics increase the chances to play well and successfully. The continuous rotation of positions, then, allows to experience different points of view of the field and to adjust to different actions companions.

Many factors come into play, such as structure and physical fitness, technical skills, tactical sense, spatial orientation, ability to predict the moves of others, ability to communicate, and understand each other and help each other in the field.

In our team, all players participate in the game: when there are more people than 12—the sum of two teams' players—we use to change a player at the time of stroke, thus allowing everyone to play. Who is not in the field at that time participates as audience. Every successful action is applauded, and people with less technical skills are strongly encouraged and applauded when they manage to keep the ball in play.

The Volleyball team regularly plays with teams of the city's high schools and participates in several tournaments during the year. In recent time, we evolved to a more engaging level of play, attending to the UISP National Championship.

5. Results and discussion

Exercise, physical activity, sports, health, mental health, psychosis, and therapy: how do these concepts relate each other? Physical activity, health, and quality of life are closely interconnected [15]; to practice sport with friends, colleagues or family do have a positive effect increasing social asset [16]. On these issues, there is a common consensus, so that Regions and States define policies to encourage physical activity. It is also generally acknowledged the positive effect of exercise on mental health, in particular on self-esteem and mood, but it is not clear whether carry it out in the open air is a further advantage; greenspaces of high natural and heritage value seem to add an extra benefit [17].

In severe psychiatric patients, exercise seems to produce an improvement in the symptoms both positive and negative [18] and quality of life [19]; in some individuals, exercise may be a useful coping strategy for dealing with positive symptoms, such as auditory hallucinations; moreover, it seems to associate with an alleviation of negative symptoms such as depression, low self-esteem, and social withdrawal. Aerobic exercise positively affects cognitive performance in hospitalized subjects, suffering from schizophrenia or depression [20]. Physical activity in severe psychiatric disorders helps to prevent metabolic and cardiovascular diseases [21], improves the satisfaction about the body and self-esteem [22], and is used as part of a multifunctional rehabilitation treatment in schizophrenia, although the negative symptoms may hinder the program, reducing the motivation and causing dropouts [23]. The exercise of an overlearned physical skill, as biking, improves brain connectivity in patients and healthy individuals [24]. While in the review by Patel [25] on a wide range of mental disorders, the effects on schizophrenia are defined as "not known," the review of Soundy et al. [26] lists the possible benefits of sports activities in this disorder, and the Firth et al.'s review [27] concludes that a moderate to vigorous exercise for about 90 min per week has a therapeutic effect by decreasing cardiovascular risk factors and reducing the psychic symptoms.

The literature offers heterogeneous works, using a wide range of exercise (aerobic, anaerobic, sports) in different contexts (inpatients and outpatients), with fairly short follow-up times and limited samples; currently, it is not possible to generalize the results, or choose an activity over another, only according to the literature.

Physical activity, exercise, sport are they synonymous? In our opinion, they are not. Physical activity and exercise, at least how they are described in many works, pose as major goals the physical muscular mobilization and the cardio-vascular prevention. The concept of sport, in our view, is different: it means to deal freely with rules shared by all those who practice it, healthy or sick; it means trying to play technically or with a good performance, in a controlled environment, aiming to improve. It means, in team sports, interfacing with peers and with opponents and dealing with mistakes and defeats as part of the game. Finally, it means tackling success without humiliating opponents. Sports are leisure activities, strictly linked to concepts such as fun and enjoyment, which also constitute the main motivation to maintain the practice [28, 29].

Can a person with schizophrenic disorders deal with all it? If it does, may he/she encounter difficulties and advantages that can face? In summary, what are the specific therapeutic factors? The literature indicates the presence, in the schizophrenia spectrum disorders, of both neurocognitive deficits and social cognition deficits, related to each other but not overlapping. The neurocognitive deficits have a role in influencing the "functional outcome": self and interpersonal behaviors and skills for independent life; they can concern attention, short or long-term memory and the ability to solve problems. The Social Cognition concerns empathy, the ability to recognize and understand emotions and feelings of others, and also the ability to infer intentions, beliefs and desires of other people [30–32].

Cognitive deficits appear related to negative symptoms and a poor functional outcome: being able to modulate the functions of social cognition may be an important factor in determining the outcome of the disease and in promoting a full recovery [33]. Sport can be one of the strategies.

Sport can be one of the strategies to improve both neurocognitive aspects and social cognitive abilities. In this context, Corretti et al. [34] propose sports as a useful tool in every stage of the disease: pre-acute, post-acute and even chronic.

From our point of view, that of an users' association, we have no direct information on the effects of exercise or sport on the pathogenesis of schizophrenia: our intervention begins when the disease is overt, when there is already a diagnosis and a therapeutic program.

http://dx.doi.org/10.5772/65632

Our experience confirms some literature data: some of our athletes report that the sport has provided them some tools to better cope with symptoms as hallucinations, especially auditory: to fix the attention on other bodily perceptions, or on the current game in team sports, antagonizes hallucinations and decreases their disturbing effect. In team sports, the habit to trust others and the self-esteem improvement are effective antagonists of some delusions, particularly those of persecution.

5.1. The users' point of view

In over 15 years of sporting activities in the area of psychiatric disorders, especially schizophrenia, we have accumulated a wealth of experience. After several interviews with our users/athletes, we would like to try to use their words to a "collective" description of their experience in the disease, and subsequently in sport.

5.1.1. The experience of illness

When you get sick of schizophrenia, the world falls upon you: everything is confused, your head is filled up with noise, you do not recognize the person you were before and even your environment; you do not know who to trust in. Above all, you do not know what is happening to you.

Family members and friends see you strange, they eventually could think that you take substances (sometimes, it is true), but the strangeness remains even when you are "clean". Some people pity you or are ashamed of you; sometimes they get angry and you get angry too. No one knows what to do.

Sooner or later you obtain a diagnosis and someone takes charge of you. Therapy begins: at least, the radio in your head lowers the volume, maybe turns off, but you have to deal with the medicines every day: now you are, first of all, a sick! Sometimes therapies bother, to find the right dose and the right drug is not always easy; sometimes you're too sedated and you look like a zombie, sometimes you get fat and bloated, or stiff and walking like a robot, or your hands and your mouth shake. Everything is treatable, but in the meantime you seem even stranger.

Your family members begin to protect you a bit too much, to treat you like when you were thirteen. Sometimes, they think you are doing it on purpose, that you spoil the situation, that you don't help yourself enough. Even to pronounce the name of the disease is very difficult: it is better to talk about "depression" or "nervous exhaustion": people can understand it. And you wish to have another illness instead of this, any: a broken leg, pneumonia, anything but that.

You start to look for the "guilty" of illness: another disease, a sentimental disappointment, a lack of work, a failure in the studies. Sometimes you think that the diagnosis is wrong, the doctor is incompetent, and "the pilgrimage of hope" begins, towards more and more well-known and expensive doctors or faraway places, where perhaps a miracle will happen.

In all this, you become more and more passive, and more and more really depressed: ill, chronically, considered untreatable, you feel useless and you hide from previous friends and you run out of your previous life, so that no one could see how much you are changed. Only in your room you feel safe, even in the dark and with the music on headphones. Even complaining does not work: there is always someone who does that before and more of you.

Every business and social relationship loses its meaning, the sense of emptiness is spreading, it is difficult to express in words. It seems that nothing interests you, even if, within you, emotions and fears are pressing. It's hard to pay attention, to decode the expressions of others people: you search isolation so not to be injured. If in your life "before" there were plans, expectations, hopes, now, in the limbo of disease, the idea prevails that everything will always be the same, or rather will only worsen.

Sometimes we get stubborn, but then we accept to follow a therapeutic process where everything is very structured and encoded and disease-related: it continually reminds us of the disease. There is not much room for fun or for personal initiatives, but then, when we have to go outside in real - not protected - world, there we must to walk alone.

5.1.2. The experience in sports

Soft gymnastic is often considered mostly as exercise, whereas all other activities are considered and lived as sports. All interviewed user-athletes expressed a positive opinion: they are happy to play sports and think it is a useful tool for them both physically and psychologically. All users emphasize the importance of working together within a group, also in individual activities, and find a good social environment, which allowed the development of better social relationships and friendships.

The main reported benefits of gymnastics and swimming are to improve agility and muscle coordination, to reach a greater satisfaction with the own body and a feeling of well-being; in swimming, they are also enhanced by learning new skills and improve self-esteem overcoming fears. In team sports, the main positive aspects are fun and the feeling of belonging, in addition to the opportunities for tournaments. The rare reported difficulties are in football, for the management of aggressiveness. In volleyball, there is a great sense of teamwork and pride for the ability to face and overcome obstacles and the ethical and educational values of which the team is witness. There is a general demand for a more frequent activity, as a source of great personal satisfaction and good social relations.

All athletes emphasize that, when they are within the sport, they completely dismiss the sick role, and they feel only people, citizens and especially athletes. This allows them to improve their self-esteem, and even increase in value with respect to the family and the environment.

5.2. The role of sport in the therapeutic project

What needs can be met in the sport, and what are consequently the objectives? Well-being, skills, to avoid isolation, to build activities for leisure, to deal with other people, to improve self-esteem and quality of life, to acquire autonomy. The different activities offer varied opportunities and have different indications and features.

Gymnastics, for example, can be a preparatory: a good start for those who do not move since a long time and have to learn to well perceive their body. It is a good motivation to leave the house, and does not require an excessive involvement in social relations, although it provides the opportunity. For people who continue to practice, it is a useful tool for physical well-being, posture, equilibrium, self-knowledge and anxiety management.

In swimming, the more specific aspects are weightless and floating: it should be interesting a further investigation about the specific effects of various bodily perceptions in the aquatic environment and their effect on body image and on perception system in general, so often impaired in schizophrenia. The acquisition of new skills and the achievement of objectives increase self-esteem, while the informal moments can provide a "play area" that allows exercising relational skills.

Football, the most popular sport in the country, both as a practice and as interest of individuals and the media, is also the one who, in the literature, seems to receive particular attention as a therapeutic rehabilitative tool. Battaglia et al. [35] studies football as an additional treatment in schizophrenia, and Masala et al. [36] describes a training protocol for football in this syndrome. Football, however, forces us to reflect on the significance of sport: it affects huge economic interest; the overpaid players, very popular, can convey positive social values but also negative. Some famous players often express in the field behaviors that would be considered highly symptomatic of mental disorder, off the field. Intolerant, provocative, threatening, aggressive, simulators; in the face of all this, they are not strongly discouraged, recalled or punished. Admonitions, expulsions and disqualifications, but then they come back and behave exactly the same way. There are matches that look like gladiator fights: faults, yellow cards, expulsions and all players exaggerate the effects of contrasts; in the meanwhile, speakers repeatedly define the game with adjectives like "hard," "aggressive," "male," all presented as positive and praiseworthy. Some fans, then, go to see football as if they were going to a battle: framed in organized groups, often armed with assault weapons, ready to destroy "the enemy" and everything they find on their way.

How can we reconcile these dis-dominant values with a sport practiced in view of psychiatric rehabilitation, with ethical and educational values? It is not always easy: there is a conflict. Almost all football teams we know were faced with this difficulty: some of them have found strategies to deal with it, others (especially ones inside the Psychiatric Services) preferred to channel the energies on other sports. We are however convinced that aggressiveness challenge can be addressed and overcome. That indeed is one of the most important goals of our activity: to learn how to deal with our and others' aggressiveness and overcome it. When we play in schools, one of our goals, in addition to combating the stigma, is to give a good example of an ethical and educational way to play the game of football.

In his very interesting and documented work, Carboni [37] defines the football as "a cognitive gym" useful to reach psychosocial health goals. For us, this happens especially with the volleyball, the sport that gives us most satisfaction, the one where you go to training half an hour before, and later you stay there chatting, joking, and making plans with your playmates and friends. It is our "cognitive fitness," this sport easy to learn, good looking, flexible respect to the number of players, cheap because you can play almost anywhere, even in the public gardens and on the beach. Few experiences are reported in the international literature, but they all are very positive [38, 39], even in the adapted version of sitting volley [40].

The volleyball allows improving a lot of cognitive skills: attention, spatial orientation, perception and recognition of a range of situations, decision-making skills, strategy: it is a problem-solving training in a context of play, which fully satisfies the Rasmussen general pattern of human activity [41].

"Was I wrong?" "Have the others been better or smarter than us?" "No problem, try again and see if it works, with a new strategy, or even the same as before, but better applied." It is no coincidence that the tradition of the game suggests to newly serve the player who has made a mistake, in order to give him/her the opportunity to rebuild and regain confidence. Point after point, play after play, self-esteem and ability to cope with the emotions grow together with the sense of the group-team. The players reflect one each other as in a mirror; following the mirror neurons theory [42], this means to communicate and to understand each other better and better. Meanwhile, people get used to work in an organized way, to come out from the isolation and to look around: it really means a training for life.

5.3. Outcomes

5.3.1. How is effectiveness measured?

A first indicator may be the number of hospitalizations: people practicing physical and sport activities require fewer hospitalizations than when they were inactive; some people decreased from 4 to 5 annual admissions to one or none. During the past year, in the group of users athletes there were only four admissions: one in the ward for acute symptoms, which lasted 2 weeks, and three, in three different people, in facilities for intensive rehabilitation programs.

A second indicator may be the adhesion to the treatment in general and, in particular, to sport classes. We do not remember, in the last 5 years, the necessity of Compulsory Admissions in people who attend sports groups; in our opinion, this means that users become more aware of their own care and they are more participating and reliable in applying it. The drop-out in sport activity is rare, usually due to external causes: family burdens, work activities, physical illness or injury. Often the injured or convalescent athletes will participate to the gym classes, to cheer their friends and even to play a useful role as "external" observers.

A third indicator is the user-athletes satisfaction and their families: sport activity is very appreciated by the family for the promotion of personal autonomy, independence and for its socializing value.

Even high school students really appreciate the opportunity to play against our teams, and their teachers feel these activities as very qualifying and deeply educational.

An external observation is provided by the interviewed referees: they all highlight the fair play of MHD teams. Furthermore, they describe a feature that makes us very happy: they knew nothing, before, of mental disorders, they expected to referee matches of very low level, and they were pleasantly surprised to find a good knowledge of the rules, a decent technical level, a pleasant game, surrounded by a great enthusiasm.

5.3.2. Quality of life

The perceived quality of life was measured in the group of users athletes, 51 people, 30 males and 21 females using the WHOQOL-brief scale 26 items. All schedules are valid.

The overall quality of life is perceived in all cases as "good" or "very good" and only 12% of people are dissatisfied with their own health.

The level of physical perceived health is high: the majority of cases declare that they feel well, without pain, full of energy, able to cope with their daily activities; many people have a job. They need some treatment, but they don't consider this as an impairment.

Psychological health level is high, too: only 6 people are unhappy about their appearance, they are mainly self-satisfied and able to concentrate. The majority think that life is pleasant and meaningful. None of the athletes-users felt always or often discouraged, in the last few months.

Information, mobility, safe and security, place where they live and transport does not show any kind of dissatisfaction or problem, but the financial resources are very limited, just enough to cover the needs, in 65% of cases; it is difficult to engage in leisure activities for a lack of money and time.

They are very satisfied for the support received from friends, quite satisfied about their personal relationships, often unsatisfied in the sexual activities area.

Overall, the perceived Quality of Life looks good and it is very significant that it is also good in the Domains most at risk in schizophrenia: Social Relationships and Psychological Aspects.

6. Conclusion

Sport is a universal language, recognized and shared by all. It promotes well-being, self-esteem and social relationships, it improves compliance and fosters an active attitude of the users/athletes; no one feels excluded.

We think that sport is a very useful and inexpensive tool in the overall frame of the treatment of schizophrenic disorders. During the first definition of the therapeutic program, sport promotes the establishment of a good relationship with the treating team and improves the adherence to treatment. It introduces the new users, especially young people, in a friendly and fun environment that helps them to overcome many misconceptions about the role of a "psychiatric patient," by seeing other people, who are users and athletes, well integrated into society. Moreover, it is an appropriate form of secondary prevention against chronic medical conditions related to sedentariness, avoiding weight gain and its deleterious effects on health, quality of life, general functioning and compliance.

In a subsequent period, it becomes targeted to specific needs of individual cases and assumes a greater significance as an effective tool for psychiatric rehabilitation, easy to implement and inexpensive. It can reduce the hospitalizations, improve Social Functioning, achieve a good quality of life, promote social inclusion and functional recovery. Schizophrenia is not a malignant disease that inevitably deteriorates over time [43]: we must work to promote recovery in every single person.

Sport allows gradually regaining a role in a social environment and finding a life domain where the disease remains outside. In our opinion, team sports have a high therapeutic value. The team is not a sum of individuals, but a unique "entity." In an ideal society, the individuals fade away and the players become a "single body" whose parts interact each other. The stronger parts support the weaker parts; the resources of all are at stake and enhanced to create that Universe-Group which aims to get the best result. Play on a team means to know and apply the rules of the sport, find the correct position on the field, learn and use specific technical skills, collaborate with others, respect fellow and opponents. The victory is a moment of cohesion and sharing of positive emotion: the result of everyone's work; even the defeat, though, is constructive, producing reflection and the reorganization of the work of the team. It is not a rewarding experience, but it's definitely a growth factor and analysis: sport teaches us to accept failures as part of a learning process or as one of the factors of the game.

Fitness, technical skills, attention, observation skills, and willingness to cooperate: these are all important factors and build expertise and resources that, if exploited, give a role in the team and increase self-esteem. Within the teams, valid relationships can grow and continue beyond the classes, producing autonomous leisure opportunities.

In our opinion, sport "treatment" combines the features of the clinical work, of clinical research and of self-help systems. We think that the treatment of schizophrenia requires a personalized approach, which evaluates the characteristics and needs of each individual: this also applies to exercise and sport: we always prefer the concept of "sport" to that of "exercise," for its value on self-esteem and social integration. In our experience of users, we suggest starting out, especially in the post-acute phase, with the proposal to an individual activity such as gymnastics, allowing a period of observation and adaptation to the movement in a friendly but not too-demanding environment. Subsequently, we propose to try an additional sport, according to the therapeutic needs and preferences of the individual subject; after an initial phase of welcome, the user will continue to practice weekly, at least for a year. Many users continue to practice sports for years, when they are symptoms-free and also after finishing their course of treatment, as volunteers.

Our and others experiences using sport in the treatment of schizophrenia may act as suggestion and encouragement toward a research centered on outpatients, using shared outcome indicators and providing for a sufficiently long follow-up, to evaluate the persistency of benefits over time. It would be very interesting also to carry out research on the different sports and on their various potentially therapeutic factors.

http://dx.doi.org/10.5772/65632

Acknowledgements

We would like to thank Enrico Balestra, president of UISP Ferrara, Gianluca Biagini, head of Volleyball UISP, Stefano Bruni, UISP swimming instructor, Giada De Biaggi, UISP volley co-instructor and Simone Merli, Councilor for Sports of the Municipality of Ferrara, for their interest and their willingness to our activity. Many thanks also to Alberto Ricci, volleyball referee, for having conceived and conducted interviews with referees.

Author details

Maria Cristina Turola[1*], Davide Barbieri[1], Angelo Palazzi[1], Veronica Pallotta[2], Luciana Simani[1,3], Chiara Tosi[1] and Ombretta Zanardi[1]

*Address all correspondence to: chiartur@gmail.com

1 Club Integriamoci NGO Association, Ferrara, Italy

2 UISP—Italian Union Sport for All, Ferrara, Italy

3 Mental Health Department—Local Health Agency, Ferrara, Italy

References

[1] Ruggeri M, Bonetto C, Lasalvia A, De Girolamo G, Fioritti A, Rucci P et al. A multi-element psychosocial intervention for early psychosis (GET UP PIANO TRIAL) conducted in a catchment area of 10 million inhabitants: study protocol for a pragmatic cluster randomized controlled trial. Trials, 2012; 13(1): 1. doi:10.1186/1745-6215-13-73

[2] Turola MC, Comellini G, Galuppi A, Nanni MG, Carantoni E, Scapoli C. Schizophrenia in real life: courses, symptoms and functioning in an Italian population. Int. J. Ment. Health. Syst., 2012; 6(1): 1. doi:10.1186/1752-4458-6-22.

[3] Overall JE, Girham DR. The brief psychiatric rating scale. Psychol. Rep., 1961; 10: 799–812.

[4] Morosini P, Magliano L, Brambilla L, Ugolini S, Pioli R. Development, reliability and acceptability of a new version of the DSM-IV Social and Occupational Functioning Assessment Scale (SOFAS) to assess routine social functioning. Acta Psychiatr. Scand., 2000; 101: 323–329.

[5] World Health Organization. "WHOQOL-BRIEF: introduction, administration, scoring and generic version of the assessment: field trial version, December 1996." Available from: www.who.int/mental_health/media/en/76.pdf [Accessed: 25-07-2016].

[6] http://sportchangeslife.com/newsstory/A_Tribute_to_Nelson_Mandela [Accessed: 24-09-2016].

[7] Isidori E. Filosofia dell'educazione sportiva. 1st ed. Roma: Editrice Nuova Cultura; 2012. (Italian)

[8] McFee G. Sport, Rules and Values. London: Routledge; 2004.

[9] http://ec.europa.eu/sport/library/policy_documents/eu-physical-activity-guidelines-2008_en.pdf [Accessed: 24-09-2016]

[10] https://www.facebook.com/IFAPA.tips/ [Accessed: 24-09-2016].

[11] https://en.wikipedia.org/wiki/Paralympic_Games [Accessed: 24-09-2016].

[12] Alexander G. Brieghel-Muller G. Eutonie. Psychol. Med., 1982; 14(6): 91–913 (French).

[13] Bertherat T,Bernstein C. The body has its reasons: anti-exercises and self-awareness. Rochester, Healing Art Press, 1989.

[14] Rywerant Y, Feldenkrais M. The Feldenkrais Method: Teaching by Handling. North Bergen, NJ: Basic Health Publications Inc.; 2003.

[15] Stewart AL, Hays RD, Wells KB, Rogers WH, Spritzer KL, Greenfield S. Long-term functioning and well-being outcomes associated with physical activity and exercise in patients with chronic conditions in the Medical Outcomes Study. J. Clin. Epidemiol., 1994; 47(7): 719–730.

[16] Coalter F. Sports clubs, social capital and social regeneration: ill-defined interventions with hard to follow outcomes? Sport Soc., 2007; 10(4): 537–559.

[17] Pretty J, Peacock J, Sellens M, Griffin M. The mental and physical health outcomes of green exercise. Int. J. Environ. Health Res., 2005; 15(5): 319–337.

[18] Guy E, Faulkner J, Taylor AH, editors. Exercise, Health and Mental Health: Emerging Relationships. 1st edition. New York: Routledge; 2005.

[19] Alexandratos K, Barnett F, Thomas Y. The impact of exercise on the mental health and quality of life of people with severe mental illness: a critical review. Br. J. Occup. Ther., 2012; 75(2): 48–60. doi:10.4276/030802212X13286281650956

[20] Oertel-Knöchel V, Mehler P, Thiel C, Steinbrecher K, Malchow B, Tesky V and Al. Effects of aerobic exercise on cognitive performance and individual psychopathology in depressive and schizophrenia patients. Eur. Arch. Psychiatry Clin. Neurosci., 2014; 264(7): 589–604. doi:10.1007/s00406-014-0485-9.

[21] Richardson CR, Faulkner G, McDevitt J, Skrinar GS, Hutchinson DS et al. Integrating physical activity into mental health services for persons with serious mental illness. Psychiatr. Serv., 2005; 56: 324–331.

[22] Maggouritsa G, Kokaridas D, Stoforos P, Patsiaouras A, Diggelidis N, Theodorakis Y. The effect of a physical activity program on improving body cathexis and self-esteem of patients with schizophrenia. Inq. Sports Phys. Educ., 2014; 12: 40–51.

[23] Vancampfort D, De Hert M, Stubbs B, Ward PB, Rosenbaum S, Soundy A, Probst M. Negative symptoms are associated with lower autonomous motivation towards physical activity in people with schizophrenia. Compr. Psychiatry, 2015; 56: 128–132.

[24] Svatkova A, Mandl RC, Scheewe TW, Cahn W, Kahn RS, Pol HE. Physical exercise keeps the brain connected: biking increases white matter integrity in patients with schizophrenia and healthy controls. Schizophr. Bull., 2015; 41(4): 869–878.

[25] Patel S, Sumeet P, De Sousa A. Exercise and mental health: a clinical. Int. J. Sci. Res., 2013; 2(7): 360–365.

[26] Soundy A, Roskell C, Stubbs B, Probst M, Vancampfort D. Investigating the benefits of sport participation for individuals with schizophrenia: a systematic review. Psychiatr. Danub, 2015; 27(1): 2–13.

[27] Firth J, Cotter J, Elliott R, French P, Yung AR, et al. A systematic review and meta-analysis of exercise interventions in schizophrenia patients. Psychol. Med., 2015; 45(7): 1343–1361.

[28] O'Reilly E, Tompkins J, Gallant M. They ought to enjoy physical activity, you know?: struggling with fun in physical education. Sport Educ. Soc., 2001; 6(2): 211–221.

[29] Carraro A, Young MC, Robazza C. A contribution to the validation of the physical activity enjoyment scale in an Italian sample. Soc. Behav. Person, 2008; 36(7): 911–918.

[30] Green MF, Kern RS, Braff DL, Mintz J. Neurocognitive deficits and functional outcome in schizophrenia: are we measuring the" right stuff"? Schizophr. Bull., 2000; 26(1): 119–136.

[31] Couture SM, Penn DL, Roberts DL. The functional significance of social cognition in schizophrenia: a review. Schizophr. Bull., 2006; 32(suppl): S44–S63.

[32] Garety PA, Bebbington P, Fowler D, Freeman D, Kuipers E. Implications for neurobiological research of cognitive models of psychosis: a theoretical paper. Psychol. Med., 2007; 37(10): 1377–1391.

[33] De Risio A. Social Cognition and Outcome. In: Tomiki Sumiyoshi, editor. Schizophrenia Research: Recent Advances. New York: Nova Science Publishers; 2012.

[34] Corretti G, Martini C, Greco PL, Marchetti FP. Sport in psychiatric rehabilitation: a tool in pre-acute, post-acute and chronic phase. Int. J. Clin. Med., 2011; 2:568–569. doi: 10.4236/ijcm.2011.25093.

[35] Battaglia G, Alesi M, Inguglia M, Roccella M, Caramazza G, Bellafiore M, Palma A. Soccer practice as an add-on treatment in the management of individuals with a diagnosis of schizophrenia. Neuropsychiatr. Dis. Treat., 2013; 9: 595–603.

[36] Masala D, Giangiuliani M, Minatrini D, Vinci G. Protocol of physical and technical-tactical training in football for schizophrenic patients. Senses Sci., 2014; 1(2): 73–76. doi: 10.14616/sands-2014-2-7376.

[37] Carboni V. Il football come palestra di atteggiamenti. Medico e bambino, 2001; 1: 60–64 (Italian).

[38] http://www.sfnsw.org.au/MHSN/Sports/mhsn-Volleyball#.V-YqGPmLTIV [Accessed: 24-09-2016]

[39] www.imsmagazine.com/volleyball-without-stigma/ page 41 [Accessed: 24-09-2016]

[40] Ćorić O, Ljubotina D. Life quality of war veterans with physical disabilities playing sitting volleyball. Ljetopis socijalnog rada, 2014; 20(3): 387–414.

[41] Rasmussen J. Skills, rules, and knowledge; signals, signs, and symbols, and other distinctions in human performance models. IEEE Trans. Syst. Man Cybern, 1983; 3: 257–266.

[42] Rizzolatti G, Fabbri-Destro M, Cattaneo L. Mirror neurons and their clinical relevance. Nat. Clin. Prac. Neurol., 2009; 5(1): 24–34.

[43] Zipursky RB, Reilly TJ, Murray RM. The myth of schizophrenia as a progressive brain disease. Schizophr. Bull., 2013; 39(6): 1363–1372.